Sing of Dignity

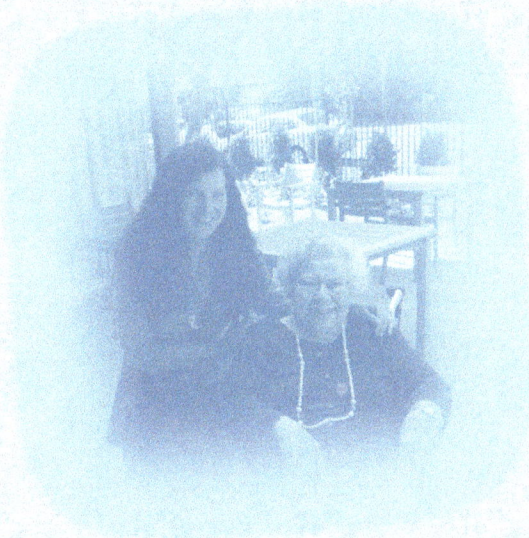

Caring at end-of-life

Dr Julie Morsillo
Community Psychologist

Sing of dignity: Caring at end-of-life

Handbook for carers of elderly – inc. dementia & palliative care

Resource Publications
An Imprint of Wipf and Stock Publishers
199 W. 8th Ave., Suite 3
Eugene, OR 97401

www.wipfandstock.com

PAPERBACK ISBN: 979-8-3852-7005-7
HARDCOVER ISBN: 979-8-3852-7006-4
EBOOK ISBN: 979-8-3852-7007-1

Previous handbooks by this author
Published by Wipf & Stock Publishers
Sing me a song to soar:
Finding hope in our redemptive stories

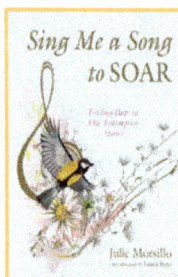

We sing songs for life:
Valuing people and the planet

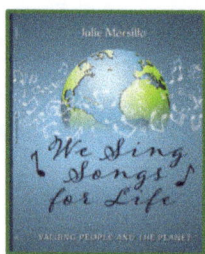

Caring for the elderly towards the end of life, can be distressing. Watching them become frail in mind and body can be heart-breaking. This handbook offers practical support and creative ideas to soothe and calm loved elderly people with dementia, towards the end of their lives, with music and reminiscence therapy. Plus, ways for those in palliative care to leave a meaningful legacy for their families and friends, with biography, narrative and dignity therapies.

Endorsements:

"This is a rare and deeply practical guide that weaves together academic insight with profound human warmth. Whether you are a professional caregiver or someone who simply loves and cares for the elderly, this book will become your steadfast companion—transforming each act of care into a moment of grace and mutual healing. I wholeheartedly recommend it to all who walk the path of elder care. This soul map deserves a permanent place on our desks, ready to be opened and rediscovered."
—**Xiaoxiao Susanna Wang**, Clinical Pastoral Care Practitioner and Counsellor

"So thankful for this handbook. It will inform and help carers to be aware of their massive impact when providing care to elderly people. It highlights the human aspect that Morsillo beautifully identifies as human dignity. Empathy is a significant element in our human interactions and relationships. I loved reading it, very easy to follow, I learnt a lot."
—**Jenn Geravito**, Pastor and Latin-American Community Worker

"Sing of Dignity: Caring at End-of-Life is the third practical narrative therapy resource book from Dr. Julie Morsillo. It provides a compassionate framework for working with people who are elderly or reaching end-of-life to provide positive closure and meaning at an otherwise difficult time."
—**Katherine Thompson**, Clinical Social Worker

"A very knowledgeable and practical handbook. I see the relevance for carers supporting loved ones through giving hope and meaning. In the counselling setting I can see how the themes and therapies can be used with a group, individual, or a workshop. Personally, I am particularly keen in encouraging hope and 'nurturing the spirit.'"
—**Amanda Roberts**, Nurture Counselling

"A great resource for families to assist in the process of grief while capturing the treasures of story, and a guide for those who are seeking a way to leave memoir and legacy for their loved ones."
—**Candy Daniels**, Founding Director, Life Wellbeing Services

"As a palliative care volunteer who has also led seminars for the elderly at my church, I appreciate the practical and helpful ways to put dignity into practice using therapies like music therapy, biography work, and narrative therapy."
—**Lili Niu**, Counsellor in English & Mandarin

"Uniting Agewell is a project I am part of, where carers and people living at home can access music. This handbook could be a great resource for the music therapist who runs the program."
—**Catriona Milne**, Educator and Social Worker

"Amazed at Julie Morsillo's insight and research for this handbook. Plus, her own practical service to the senior folk she has faithfully cared for over the years. I've watched Julie and been astounded by her consistency and understanding of each one's own particular needs."
—**Alice Jeffries**, Retired Art Teacher

"What a valuable resource this is. It all looks incredibly good, needed, helpful, practical, sensitive, and kind."
—**Angleo Cettolin,** Dean of Faculty, Eastern College Australia

"This will be a wonderful encouragement to those caring for elderly loved ones."
—**Cheryl Osment,** Academic Administrator, Eastern College Australia

"We wholeheartedly support Morsillo's efforts to benefit older adults and promote spiritual care."
—**Rachael Wass**, CEO, Meaningful Aging Australia

Introduction

Caring for the elderly towards the end of life, can be distressing. Watching them become frail in mind and body can be heart-breaking. This handbook offers practical support for those offering clinical and pastoral care to the elderly, especially people with dementia and those in palliative care towards the end of their lives. The handbook provides some guidance and resources to understand the various stages and changing behaviours of people suffering from dementia, with some practical hints on how to manage challenging times. Creative ideas to soothe and calm loved elderly people towards the end of their lives, with music and reminiscence therapy. Plus, ways for those in palliative care to leave a meaningful legacy for their families and friends, with biography, narrative and dignity therapies.

Dedication

To all the many compassionate carers who work tirelessly to care for the elderly towards the end of their lives. Many unpaid, low paid and voluntary, with little recognition or a voice of their own, giving up time and much of their own needs and dreams, to give dignity of care to their loved ones or others loved ones.

Acknowledgments

To all the elderly people of my family and my church community, whom I have offered pastoral care in the twilight years of their lives. They have taught me so much about giving compassion to others when they could, especially to those in need. Towards the end of their lives, they showed a humble gratitude for small services of care towards them. May I be as gracious and grateful, when I face the final days of my life.

Thanks to Ian Heng, who researched *End of life care and spirituality* as a Master of Community Counselling student, of Eastern College Australia, who also studied theology. His research inspired me to research this area more. Grateful for his careful referencing that I have selectively used.

Thanks to Eastern Palliative Care (Melbourne) for their work on biography therapy and allowing my counselling students to do volunteer work with them. Also, to Dignity in Care in Canada for their work on dignity therapy that this handbook draws upon so much.

Thanks to my friend Chara Meredith, for her meticulous editing. Thanks to my husband Robert, and sons Nathan and Ben, for their technical support and willingness to discuss the issues I cover in my handbooks. Thanks to my elderly mother in her 90s, Shirely Mitchell, whom I talk with daily, for her clarity of thought and encouragement of my writing projects.

Thank you all

Julie Morsillo PhD
Community Psychologist
drjulie.morsillo@gmail.com

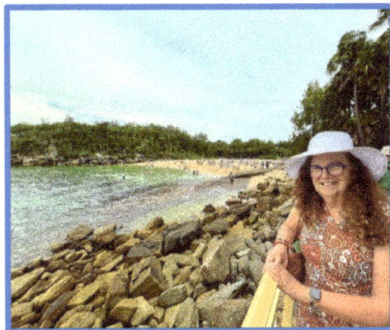

Julie at Cabbage Tree Bay,
Sydney, near where she grew up

CONTENTS

Personal Inspiration 5

PART 1: Sing of Dignity 8
1. Dignity towards elderly 8
    1.1 Dignity towards Indigenous elderly 9
    1.2 Dignity in end-of-life care 11
2. Support for Dementia 15
    2.1 Stages of dementia 16
    2.2 Dementia behaviours 18
3. Palliative caring 22
    3.1 Holistic approach 22
    3.2 Spiritual care 23

PART 2: Practice caring lullabies 24
4. Reminiscence Therapy 24
    4.1 Nostalgia 24
    4.2 Reminiscence 25
5. Music Therapy 26
    5.1 What is music therapy 26
    5.2 Benefits of music therapy in aged care 27
    5.3 Music therapy methods 30
    5.4 Sing of dignity – Music for elderly 31
6. Song of Life biographical music therapy 33
    6.1 Biographical interview..33
    6.2 Meaningful biographical song performance 33
7. Biography Therapy 34
    7.1 Biographical story recorded 34
    7.2 Meaningful story as legacy 34
8. Narrative therapy for end of life 36
    8.1 Re-membering identity 36
    8.2 Re-membering from dying mothers for their children 36
9. Dignity therapy...37
    9.1 Care with dignity...37
    9.2 Connect with dignity 37
    9.3 Communicate with dignity 38
10. Practice of dignity therapy 39
    10.1 Seek special times...39
    10.2 Knock for family photos and travels 39
    10.3 Ask for favourite music, foods & nature...40
    10.4 Love given to others 41
11. Death doula 42
12. Dealing with grief after death 45

Resources & supports 48

Personal Inspiration

End of life with my Dad

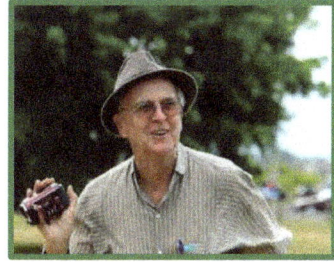

My father, Phillip Nebuchadnezzar Mitchell, known as Phil or Poppa, at 77 yrs old, was diagnosed with cancer and given six months to live in 2010. My mother, Shirley, had some nursing training when she was young so was confident that she could provide him palliative care at home. We had our family reunions with all of us four kids, a couple of us coming from interstate before he suffered too much with his cancer. We asked Dad to tell us stories from his younger days. He was happy to oblige. He had a good attitude toward the end of life. He said: *There were more projects that I wanted to do in life. But I have had more than my three score years and ten, that we are told in the bible makes for a long life. I can't complain.*

Throughout the last few months my Dad's pain was managed with morphine patches, and although there was still some discomfort, was largely under control. Over time he had less and less energy, could not eat much, and did not even want to watch TV. However, he listened to the radio and I knew he loved Christian hymns and choruses, and old Australian folk songs. He used to enjoy playing them on the piano accordion. As I child I would sing with him, and later with my sister too.

Fortunately, when Dad was in his last months, small shuffle iPods that hung around your neck (about the height and width of two fingers) had just become popular. So, I found as many Christian and folk songs that I could, and my husband put them into a play list on the iPod to give to him. All Dad had to do was press the start button, and the songs would automatically shuffle randomly and play into his ears. Dad loved it. He could stay lying in bed, propped up a little, smiling, listening to his beloved music.

Then in his final days, he was moved to a palliative care hospice. And when he started the *death rattle*, we were all called to his bedside, pastors came and prayed with him; and Mum decided we needed to sing him off. We sang a few of his favourite hymns: *Amazing Grace*, *The Old Rugged Cross* and *How Great Thou Art.* One of my brothers brought in a couple of copies of *Scripture in Song* booklets for us to sing choruses to him that he so liked. I think we sang many of the first 30 choruses, before Mum decided that might be enough. A few hours later he died peacefully, with his beloved music hopefully still ringing in his eyes.

Amazing Grace

Amazing grace how sweet the sound
That saved a wretch like me
I once was lost but now am found
Was blind but now I see.
John Newton (1772)

At Dad's funeral,
my now late sister Rosalie Joy
and I sang a duet acapella,
the gospel song:
I'll fly away.

Rest in peace Dad.

Story of Joyce

When I got to know her, Joyce, as an older softly spoken woman, was sad at losing her daughter and unable to see her grandchildren. However, a son was living with her for company, which helped.

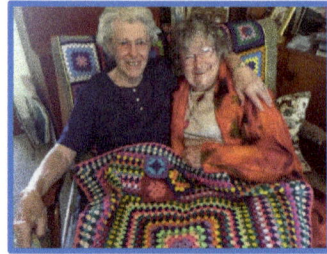
Joyce & Shirley (my Mum)

Joyce was particularly good at welcoming newcomers to our church. When Rhea, a student from the Philippines, started to come regularly to church, it was Joyce who sat with her, inviting the young woman back to her home to share lunch, play cards together, and then Joyce would drive her home.

Later, sadly, Joyce developed dementia and her son cared for her. Soon she could no longer drive or do her beloved gardening. She struggled with her crocheting of patchwork knee rugs, that she loved to make. To aid her, I would start her off with the centre part, and then she could continue making the rug grow with the repetitive patterns, using different random colours each round. When she joined the local community health centre weekly lunches at our church, for socially isolated elderly, Joyce made knee rugs for every worker who cared for her. She was a favourite.

Joyce loved her old hymns, but her eyesight was going. So I printed out the words of her two favourite hymns in large print – *Amazing Grace* and *What a Friend we have in Jesus*. She would stand near the doorway for more light, to read them and sing along with me:

However, what really got her animated was the song: *You are my sunshine, my only sunshine, you make me happy when skies are grey.* She would sing it with gusto, and point to me at the piano, every-time it came to the word '*you*'. She would dance around too, smiling gleefully.

Music was what animated her the most, near the end of her life. Her old smile would return, to light up a room, once again. You are greatly missed Joyce. Rest in peace.

Book on personal story of dementia
Still Alice by Lisa Genova, 2007, iUniverse Inc. – book and movie
Still Alice is a compelling novel about a 50-year-old woman's sudden descent into early onset Alzheimer's disease, written by first-time author Lisa Genova, who holds a PhD in neuroscience from Harvard University.

Genova, L. (2007) Still Alice. iUniverse.
Still Alice movie version – www.youtube.com/watch?v=goCp3HcT1i4

Stories to promote empathy in dementia care
The *Aging Mind Initiative*, University of Queensland, has lots of links to personal and clinical stories about people with dementia, and their carers and families. Happy reading!

Aging Mind Initiative – The University of Queensland
– https://ami.group.uq.edu.au/story-promote-empathy-dementia-care
A walk through dementia – Walking home video – Alzheimer's Research UK
– www.youtube.com/watch?v=R-Rcbj_qR4g
Dementia from the inside video – Social Care Institute for Excellence (SCIE)
– www.youtube.com/watch?v=Erjzl1WL8yQ

Seek and ye shall find
Knock and the door will be open
Ask and it shall be given
When the **love** comes trickling down

Matt 7:7-8, Gospel song by Stephen C Foster (1863)

SEEK out stories of **special times** in their lives to tell and document

KNOCK to find **photos of family and friends** to collect, label or make a photo album

ASK of favourite things to soothe, like: **music**, **food**, **nature** and favourite walks

LOVE – remembering legacy **given to others** – love to family, friends, and community

See more in section 7. Practice of Dignity Therapy

Whatsoever things are:
true
honest
just
pure
lovely
& of good report
think on these things.

Philippians 4:8

PART 1: Sing of Dignity

1. Dignity towards elderly

Dignity

forms the bedrock
of human well-being

The elderly are worthy of respect, to be treated with dignity

Dignity is a state or quality of being worthy of honour or respect.

Dignity is the quality of a person that makes them deserve respect,
sometimes shown in behaviour or appearance.

Dignity can be calm, serious and controlled behaviour
that makes people respect you.

Dignity can describe the importance and value that a person has, that makes
other people respect themselves or makes them respect themselves.

Speak up for those in need

Speak up for those who
cannot speak for themselves,
for the rights of all who are destitute.
Speak up and judge fairly;
defend the rights of the poor and needy.
Proverbs 31: 8-9

1.1 Dignity towards Indigenous elderly

The elderly are worthy of respect, to be treated with dignity

Community focused cultures, and family orientated peoples understand that the elderly of the community need to be cared for with dignity, since they are the ones who cared for us when we were young. Often in Indigenous communities around the world, the elderly are often revered, as the wise ones of the community, as they have lived through so much, and taught us so much. They leave a legacy for us.

Indigenous Australians respect elders

Australian Indigenous peoples, like other Indigenous peoples around the world, honour their elderly, who have had a lifetime of cultural learning and teaching, and are often respected with the honorary little of Aunties and Uncles of the community as an.

As an expression of respect by non-Indigenous, Indigenous Peoples of Australia, as the traditional owners of the land, and the wise elders of the communities, are often honoured with an *Acknowledgment of Country* at formal meetings and events. A traditional Indigenous ritual that continues today, is for elders of the local nation to welcome foreigners (Indigenous and non-Indigenous alike) to it by performing a *Welcome to Country*.

An Acknowledgement of Country recognises that you are meeting on the land of First Nations peoples. It's an opportunity for everyone there to show respect for Traditional Owners and their ongoing connection to Country.

> Acknowledgment of Country
>
> I'd like to acknowledge
> the traditional owners
> of the land on which we meet today.
> I would also like to pay my respects
> to elders past, present and emerging

Reconciliation Australia – www.reconciliation.org.au/reconciliation/acknowledgement-of-country-and-welcome-to-country/

Creative Spirits – Respect for elders and culture
– www.creativespirits.info/aboriginalculture/people/respect-for-elders-and-culture

Indigenous Government Australia –www.indigenous.gov.au/acknowledgement-country

Respectfully communicating with Indigenous elders in Australia – Common Ground
– www.commonground.org.au/article/guide-for-respectfully-communicating-with-elders

Yarning about aged care and your rights
– www.agedcarequality.gov.au/sites/default/files/media/yarning-about-aged-care-and-your-rights-conversation-guide.pdf

Aboriginal aged care framework
– www.health.gov.au/sites/default/files/2025-02/aboriginal-and-torres-strait-islander-aged-care-framework.pdf

Māori in New Zealand respect elders

New Zealand Māori place photos of their grandparents and their parents on the wall. Doing so, they honour their elders in their sacred long houses, as the wise ancestors of their community, who have passed on their DNA as well as their cultural stories and values to the younger generations.

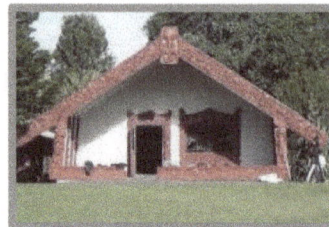

Reciprocity: Māoris Elderly and family – NZ Psychological Society – www.psychology.org.nz/journal-archive/NZJP-Vol282-1999-6-Durie.pdf

New Zealand Council of Christian Social Services – Empowerment of elderly – https://nzccss.org.nz/report/kaumatua/whakamana-empowerment/

Māori care in context

Māori *whānau* care roles, need to be understood within the dynamics of Māori notions of wellbeing, cultural roles, as well as practices related to kin relationships. Central to Māori wellbeing, is the interconnectedness of the spiritual world and material physical world. This connectedness is evident in the relationships among God, the people, and the land which confer identity and belonging. The spirits' journey from the world of potential to the worlds of becoming and of being, and return, on death, is mirrored in everyday processes and human actions.

Simpson, M.L., McAllum, K., Oetzel, J., Berryman, K., Reddy, R. (2022). Māori elders' perspectives of end-of-life family care: whānau carers as knowledge holders, weavers, and navigators. Palliative Care Social Practice. September 2022, 8;16. – https://pmc.ncbi.nlm.nih.gov/articles/PMC9459446/

African nations respect elders in community – Ubuntu

African communities honour the concept of community, Ubuntu, where the community cares for each other and learns from each other, including honouring the elders of the community.

"Where *ubuntu* flourishes, families know each other and help each other in times of crisis and need. Where *ubuntu* is present, communities are in touch with long traditions of problem solving. In a typical traditional 'ikundla' (isiZulu), or 'khotla' (Setswana), the elderly people will meet and relate the problem at hand with what has happened in the past and relate stories of relevance to the problem and find solutions. These solutions do not hurt the self-respect of the victims or perpetrators. *Ubuntu* determines that the dignity and self-respect of all must remain." (p.60).

Ubuntu

The spirit of hospitality collective trust unconditional respect dignity, racial and cultural tolerance

Kotze, E., Kotze, D., Ramantzi, L., Lebeko, C., Mafojane, S., Masondo, E., Ntshokolsha, V., & Tlhale, M. (2002). Ubuntu: Caring for people and community in South Africa – *International Journal of Narrative Therapy & Community Work,* 2002. No 1. – https://dulwichcentre.com.au/wp-content/uploads/2016/12/12-ubuntu.pdf

1.2 Dignity in end-of-life care

Dignity in care – Dr. Harvey Max Chochinov in Canada

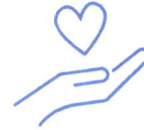

Kindness, humanity, and respect are core values of health care which must be safeguarded in our time-pressured world. Dignity in Care provides practical ideas and tools to support a culture of compassion and respect throughout the health care system.

Dignity in Care is based on 25 years of research by Dr. Harvey Max Chochinov and members of his research team, in collaboration with progressive researchers from Australia, England and the United States.

Dr. Harvey Max Chochinov, leads the research team that pioneered the Dignity Model and Dignity Therapy. Dr. Chochinov's program of research has earned him recognition as one of the world's leading palliative care scholars and researchers. He is also a Distinguished Professor of Psychiatry at the University of Manitoba, Canada. His seminal publications addressing psychosocial dimensions of palliation have helped define core-competencies and standards of upholding dignity in end-of-life care.

Findings:

- People working in health care can have a huge influence on the dignity of those who use health care services, which in turn can improve the patient experience and increase satisfaction with health care.

- Good communication is an essential ingredient for providing the best quality of health care and patient safety.

- Other researchers have found that better interactions between those who provide and use health care can result in better health outcomes for patients and improved job satisfaction for those who work in health care.

These findings show the importance of making dignity a conscious goal of health care, particularly at the bedside.

https://dignityincare.ca/en/dignity-in-care-lead-investigator.html

The Patient Dignity Question

What do I need to know
about you as a person,
to give you the best care possible?

Dignity in Care

https://dignityincare.ca/en/the-patient-dignity-question.html

More on Dignity Therapy in the second section of this handbook.

Dignity in mental healthcare

Dignity is widely recognised as a foundational concept in the provision of healthcare. Despite this, concepts of dignity are only vaguely described in the literature relating to mental health services, contributing to frequent violations of service users' dignity. Notably, discussions of dignity in mental health services often do not include the service user perspective.

A narrative review of the literature to examine how service users and peer workers articulate the co-production of dignity within mental health services, show several overarching dimensions of dignity emerge from the available evidence, spanning the:

- Social dignity that service users experience in relation with healthcare professionals
- Mental health system itself
- Physical settings in which mental health services are delivered
- Use of peers as valued members of the mental health workforce
- Peer as co-creators of knowledge.

What is dignity?

I can divide dignity into two parts. The first part is dignity within, how much dignity I feel for myself. The second part is dignity from outside, from people, government, laws and from the community…that together with inner dignity, I could live my life with pride and hope.   *Male service user*

For a **sense of wellbeing,** people in palliative care, need to feel they have:

1. Dignity of self – Human dignity in the way they see themselves – with some sense of empowerment in relation to health-care staff

2. Dignity in relation to others – in how they are perceived in relationship to others and to their setting, with some personal goals and choices within the health-care setting.

Brooks, C., Sunkel, C., & Stewart, H. L. N. (2025). Dignity in mental healthcare: Service user perspectives. *Academia Mental Health and Well-Being*, 2(1). – www.academia.edu/2997-9196/2/1/10.20935/MHealthWellB7523#B6-sustainability-3411931

NOTE: Bodily autonomy for dignity

Bodily autonomy is the ability for people who are cared for by others to maintain their right to own the decisions and ownership of their body *(bodily boundaries)* while they are alive. It is easy for carers to start to make decisions for people in their care without respecting the person's continued right to make their own decisions. It can be simple things like asking the person for permission to touch their person before doing so, allowing them to make decisions on how they want to be cared for (and not just once, every time), all the way to how politicians and policy makers get involved. Autonomy of one's own body is a form of dignity.

Lothian, K., Philp, I.(2001). Maintaining the dignity and autonomy of older people in the healthcare setting. *British Medical Journal,* 17 March 2001;322(7287), p. 668-670.

Dignity in mental health care

In a moral context, dignity is inherent in all humans and inalienable: the human worth which a person enjoys simply by virtue of being human and which cannot be lost except in death. As an intrinsic human quality, dignity is shared and acknowledged between human beings; dignity is both being *('What I am')* and the recognition of being in others. Human dignity is universally understood as part of the collective unconscious, creating an archetypal understanding across cultures of how individuals want to be perceived.

Human rights are *'specifications of human dignity'* (Habermas, 2010) and are the conduit through which abstract concepts of morality become legislation. According to human rights statutes, all humans are equal in dignity and rights, and discriminating against a person because of physical, mental or cognitive disability, is a violation of inherent dignity and human rights.

The importance of dignity as a moral concept has been widely recognized in mental healthcare professional (HCP) ethics, healthcare policy and patient experience. Yet mental healthcare services worldwide, according to the World Health Organization (WHO) and the United Nations (UN), do not respect the dignity of service users; further, stigma and the continued use of coercive practices can lead to human rights violations in mental healthcare (WHO, 2023). The contributory factors to dignity violation in mental health services are complex and include policy planning and monitoring, and limited resources to mental healthcare and services. Only 2% of global expenditure on health is spent on mental health, with just under 4% in high-income countries (HICs)

Human dignity can be described as an inherent and inalienable human quality, which is manifested as both self-respect and respect from others. Dignity flows from two separate sources: one internal (self-respect, *'how I see myself'*) and one external (respect, *'how others see me'*) in a constantly dynamic process involving both internal and external components. The *'dignified self'* has self-respect and respect from others; because self-respect is dynamic, so dignity is dynamic. This definition of dignity as *'dignity of identity'* can be enhanced or undermined by other people or situations including illness and aging.

Dignity is characterized by *'being seen'* by others; *'not being seen'* involves not being heard and acknowledged, as well as being seen only as a member of a group and not as an individual or being separated from a group or social norm, i.e. being stigmatised.

> "(I was) treated with dignity – I talked. She listened. Not only was I treated with dignity, but I was treated with warmth. I felt safe and I felt liberated of my own feelings which, until then, had been buried somewhere inside my skinny body. In this experience, I felt that I wasn't shamed for the difficulties I was facing or questioned for the things I did. This is what it feels like to be treated with dignity."
>
> *Female service user*

Brooks, C., Sunkel, C., & Stewart, H. L. N. (2025). Dignity in mental healthcare: Service user perspectives. *Academia Mental Health and Well-Being*, 2(1). – www.academia.edu/2997-9196/2/1/10.20935/MHealthWellB7523#B6-sustainability-3411931

World Health Organization (WHO). (2023). Mental health, human rights and legislation. – www.who.int/publications/i/item/9789240080737

Dignity in mental health care (continued)

Mental health represents a significant global public health issue, impacting not only affected individuals but families and societies. Perceptions of people with a mental illness often result in stigmatization, casting doubt on their capacity, intelligence, and right to take advantage of opportunities provided by the global community, denying dignity and worth. Individuals experiencing mental health concerns are often viewed as responsible for their diagnosis, suggesting a lack of knowledge regarding the etiopathology of mental illness. A positive proactive approach to stigma reduction via enhanced mental health literacy is warranted.

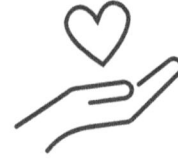

Livingston, V., Jackson-Nevels, B., Davis-Wagner, D., Jameson, D., & Joyner, C. (2025). Dignity in mental health—examining the dynamics of mental health stigma: a narrative review. *Academia Mental Health and Well-Being*, 2(3).

Dignity forms the bedrock of human well-being. It reflects our inherent worth as individuals, regardless of our mental state or health challenges. In mental health settings, dignity shows up when providers treat people with respect, protect their right to make choices, and ensure they can access quality care. Yet, despite widespread lip service to these ideals, mental health systems worldwide often fail to deliver dignity in practice. People seeking help instead encounter stigma, discrimination, inadequate services, and policies that neglect their needs Tackling these problems requires communities, healthcare workers, and policymakers to work together on multiple fronts.

Anders, R. (2025). Dignity in mental health care: human rights challenges and pathways. *Academia Mental Health and Well-Being,* 2(2).

Habermas, J. (2010) The concept of human dignity and the realistic utopia of human rights. *Metaphilosophy.* 2010;41(4):464–80.

Marley, J. A. (2005). Concept analysis of dignity. Essential Concepts of Nursing. Edinburgh: *Elsevier Churchill Livingstone,* 2005, p. 77–91.

Nordenfelt, L., & Edgar, A. (2005). The four notions of dignity. Quality Ageing. 6(1), p.17–21.

World Health Organization (WHO). (2023). Mental health, human rights and legislation – www.who.int/publications/i/item/9789240080737

"Treat people with respect.
You never know, that might be the first time they have ever been treated with respect."

The late Jan Pentland who came from the 'wrong side of the tracks' and partner David Morawetz

See: Jan Pentland Foundation – www.janpentlandfoundation.org

2. Support for Dementia

Dementia is a brain condition. It's not a normal part of ageing.

Dementia is a general term for loss of memory, language, problem-solving and other thinking abilities that are severe enough to interfere with daily life. Alzheimer's is the most common cause of dementia.

Dementia doesn't just impact the person living with the condition and their immediate carers; it also impacts their friends, family and wider social network.

2.1 Changes in behaviour

Many people living with dementia experience changes in behaviour, including:

- Anxiety or apathy
- Sleep changes
- Walking or pacing
- Distress during personal care
- Wanting to leave or go home
- Agitation or aggression
- Disinhibition
- Hallucinations

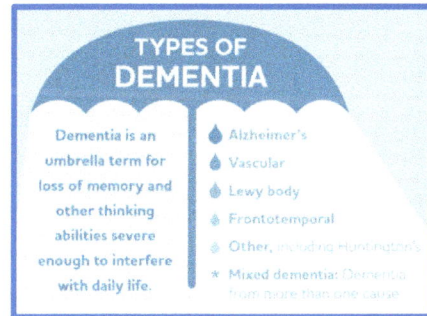

TYPES OF DEMENTIA

Dementia is an umbrella term for loss of memory and other thinking abilities severe enough to interfere with daily life.

- Alzheimer's
- Vascular
- Lewy body
- Frontotemporal
- Other, including Huntington's
- Mixed dementia: Dementia from more than one cause

There are many reasons why someone living with dementia may begin to behave differently. Physical changes in the brain affect memory, judgement, communication, and emotional regulation. However, behaviour is also shaped by a person's environment and experiences.

Pain, discomfort, confusion, overstimulation, fatigue, or unmet needs, even something as simple as hunger or needing the toilet, can all influence behaviour. Changes in routine or surroundings may also contribute. For many people living with dementia, behaviour becomes a primary way of communicating when words are no longer easy to find.

It's important to understand that behaviours such as anxiety, agitation, aggression, or social withdrawal are not intentional. They are signals that the person may be feeling distressed, overwhelmed, unsafe or unsure of what is happening around them. Though these moments can be difficult and at times upsetting, an empathetic approach can make a significant difference — both for the person living with dementia and their carers.

The carer handbook for understanding changed behaviours
Dementia Support Australia – www.dementia.com.au

See also: **Australian Government supports for carers**
www.servicesaustralia.gov.au/getting-support-if-youre-caring-for-someone?context=60097
and Carer Gateway – www.carergateway.gov.au

NOTE: Elderly migrants often revert to language of origin

Hanna, F. (2025). For migrants' dementia can mean losing a language and a whole world. *The Conversation.* 12 September 2025. https://theconversation.com/for-migrants-dementia-can-mean-losing-a-language-and-a-whole-world-263185

15

2.1   Stages of dementia

Early stage – mild

A person may function independently. He or she may still drive, work and be part of social activities. Despite this, the person may feel as if he or she is having memory lapses, such as forgetting familiar words or the location of everyday objects.

Symptoms may not be widely apparent at this stage, but family and close friends may take notice and a doctor would be able to identify symptoms using certain diagnostic tools.

Common difficulties include:

- Coming up with the right word or name
- Remembering names when introduced to new people
- Having difficulty performing tasks in social or work settings
- Forgetting material that was just read
- Losing or misplacing a valuable object
- Experiencing increased trouble with planning or organizing

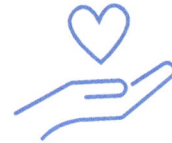

Middle stage – moderate

Middle-stage Alzheimer's is typically the longest stage and can last for many years, with the person requiring more assistance. Symptoms, which vary from person to person, may include:

- Being forgetful of events or personal history
- Feeling moody or withdrawn, especially in socially or mentally challenging situations
- Being unable to recall information about themselves like their address or telephone number, and the high school or college they attended
- Experiencing confusion about where they are or what day it is
- Requiring help choosing proper clothing for the season or the occasion
- Having trouble controlling their bladder and bowels
- Experiencing changes in sleep patterns, such as sleeping during the day and becoming restless at night
- Showing an increased tendency to wander and become lost
- Demonstrating personality and behavioural changes, including suspiciousness and delusions or compulsive, repetitive behaviour like hand-wringing or tissue shredding

In the middle stage, the person living with Alzheimer's can still participate in daily activities with assistance. It's important to find out what the person can still do or find ways to simplify tasks. As the need for more intensive care increases, caregivers may want to consider respite care or an adult day centre so they can have a temporary break from caregiving while the person living with Alzheimer's continues to receive care in a safe environment.

Alzheimer's Association – www.alz.org/alzheimers-dementia/stages

Late-stage Alzheimer's – severe

In the final stage of the disease, dementia symptoms are severe. Individuals lose the ability to respond to their environment, to carry on a conversation and, eventually, to control movement. They may still say words or phrases, but communicating pain becomes difficult. As memory and cognitive skills continue to worsen, significant personality changes may take place and individuals need extensive care.

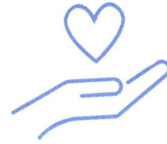

At this stage, individuals may:

- Require around-the-clock assistance with daily personal care

- Lose awareness of recent experiences as well as of their surroundings

- Experience changes in physical abilities, including walking, sitting and, eventually, swallowing

- Have difficulty communicating

- Become vulnerable to infections, especially pneumonia

The person living with Alzheimer's may not be able to initiate engagement as much during the late stage, but he or she can still benefit from interaction in ways that are appropriate, like listening to relaxing music or receiving reassurance through gentle touch. During this stage, caregivers may want to use support services, such as hospice care, which focus on providing comfort and dignity at the end of life. Hospice can be of great benefit to people in the final stages of Alzheimer's and other dementias and their families.

Alzheimer's Association – www.alz.org/alzheimers-dementia/stages

Stages of dementia video – Answers About Alzheimer's
– www.youtube.com/watch?app=desktop&v=0PBmnVb1Z9Y

Dementia Australia – www.dementia.org.au/

Dementia Support Australia. (2025). *The carer handbook for understanding changed behaviours* – www.dementia.com.au

NOTE: Younger onset dementia

Dementia Australia has a compressive handbook for anyone: diagnosed before the age of 65; carers; and family. Younger onset dementia can have significant extra challenges.

The younger onset dementia guide
– www.dementia.org.au/about-dementia/younger-onset-dementia/younger-onset-dementia-guide#download-the-younger-onset-dementia-guide

2.2   Dementia behaviours

Sundowning – late day confusion

Some of the different behaviours exhibited by those with dementia, can be affronting and distressing for the family and carers. Late day confusion is one of them.

The term *'sundowning'* refers to a state of confusion that occurs in the late afternoon and lasts into the night. Sundowning can cause various behaviours, such as confusion, anxiety, aggression or ignoring directions. Sundowning also can lead to pacing or wandering.

Sundowning isn't a disease, but a group of symptoms that occurs at a specific time of the day, that can affect people with dementia. The exact cause of sundowning is not known.

Factors that may worsen late-day confusion
- Fatigue
- Spending a day in a place that's not familiar
- Low lighting, Increased shadows
- Disruption of the body's *'internal clock'*
- Trouble separating reality from dreams
- Being hungry or thirsty
- Presence of an infection, such as a urinary tract infection
- Being bored or in pain, depression

Tips for reducing sundowning
- Keep a predictable routine for bedtime, waking, meals and activities
- Plan for activities and exposure to light during the day to support nighttime sleepiness
- Limit daytime napping
- Limit caffeine and sugar to morning hours
- Turn on a night light to reduce agitation that occurs when surroundings are dark or not familiar
- In the evening, try to reduce background noise and stimulation, includes TV viewing
- In a strange or not familiar setting, bring familiar items, such as photographs, to help relax
- In the evening, play familiar, gentle music or relaxing sounds of nature, such as the sound of waves

Some research suggests that a low dose of melatonin may help ease sundowning. Melatonin is a naturally occurring hormone that induces sleepiness. It can help when taken alone or in combination with exposure to bright light during the day.

It's possible that a medicine side effect, pain, depression or other condition could contribute to sundowning. Talk with a healthcare professional if you suspect that a condition might be making someone's sundowning worse. A urinary tract infection or sleep apnoea could be contributing to sundowning, especially if it comes on quickly.

Mayo Clinic – www.mayoclinic.org/diseases-conditions/alzheimers-disease/expert-answers/sundowning/faq-20058511
Dementia and sundowning video – Answers About Alzheimer's
– www.youtube.com/watch?app=desktop&v=UrfR3OTOBIo

Dementia Wandering and hiding

A distressing behaviour, due to safety concerns is wandering and hiding. It's common for people living with dementia to wander. This can be confusing and frightening for both the person with dementia and the carers.

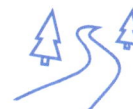

Causes of wandering

Because dementia can affect someone's memory and ability to communicate, they may not be able to tell you why they are wandering. However, these are some common reasons.

- **Memory loss:** They might set off to go to the shop or visit a friend, then forget what they were doing or where they were going.

- **Finding or doing something from their past:** They might be looking for someone or something from their past, such as a partner who has died. Or they might believe they need to do a task from their old routine, like going to work.

- **Confusion about where they are:** If they've moved house or joined a new day care centre, they might feel lost or uncertain about where they are, causing them to wander.

- **Night-time confusion:** People with dementia may wake up at night and become disoriented. They might think it is daytime and decide to go for a walk outside. Or they might believe a dream is real and respond to it.

- **Boredom or too much energy:** Wandering might be a sign that they're bored or they're not getting enough exercise during the day.

- **Agitation:** Dementia can cause people to feel restless or agitated, leading to pacing or wandering.

- **Feeling uncomfortable:** They might be wandering because they're in pain, their clothes are too hot or tight, or they need to go to the toilet. They might also be trying to escape somewhere that's too loud or busy.

- **Continuing a habit:** If they used to enjoy walking, they might want to keep doing this.

Reducing wandering

You can try to prevent or reduce wandering by:

- Visiting the doctor to check whether illness, pain or medication might be causing the wandering

- Keeping track of their wandering through a diary or log, as this can help you to work out any patterns or triggers. For example, they might wander at a specific time of the day

- Removing objects that might remind them to wander, such as handbags, coats, mail that needs posting and work clothes

- Making it more difficult for them to wander. For example, you might move the door locks or add a buzzer that makes a sound when the door opens

- Checking their clothes are comfortable

- Making sure they have familiar items around them, particularly if they've moved house recently

- Giving them a safe place to walk.

Dementia Australia
– www.dementia.org.au/living-dementia/mood-and-behaviour-changes/wandering

19

Rummaging & hiding

Another unusual behaviour of someone with dementia, is that they may start rummaging or searching through cabinets, drawers, closets, the refrigerator, and other places where things are stored. They may also hide items around the house.

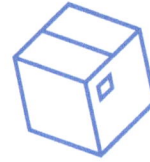

In some cases, there might be a logical reason for this behaviour. For instance, they may be looking for something specific but not able to tell you what it is. They may be hungry or bored. Try to understand what is causing the behaviour so you can fit your response to the cause.

Safer rummaging

You can take steps that allow the person with Alzheimer's to rummage while keeping the person safe. Try these tips:

- Lock up dangerous or toxic products or place them out of the person's sight and reach.

- Remove spoiled food from the refrigerator and cabinets. Someone with Alzheimer's may look for snacks but lack the judgment or sense of taste, to stay away from foods that have gone bad.

- Remove valuable items that could be misplaced or hidden by the person, such as important papers, credit cards, jewellery, mobiles, and keys.

- People with dementia often hide, lose, or throw away mail. If this is a serious problem, consider getting a post office box. If you have a yard with a fence and a locked gate, place your mailbox outside the gate.

National Institute of Ageing, USA – www.nia.nih.gov/health/alzheimers-changes-behavior-and-communication/coping-alzheimers-behaviors-rummaging-and

Why do people with dementia pack up and hide clothes video – Creative Connections in Dementia Care – www.youtube.com/watch?v=LJJhU9RuJmY

More on dementia and engagement

Elder dementia and engagement using zoom
– https://meaningfulageing.org.au/product/dementia-engagement-zoom/

More resources on caring for the elderly, including dementia

Meaningful Ageing Australia
– https://meaningfulageing.org.au/products-services/

DEMENTIA care – hints for family, friends & carers

Family and carers need to accept the new reality of the person with dementia, by not become frustrated when they have trouble remembering things or explaining things.

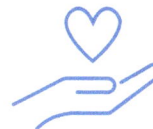

For example, it is much more helpful to announce your name on arrival when visiting someone with dementia, rather than ask them: '*Do you know who I am?*'. They can get frustrated trying to remember names and places and explain what their needs are.

However, you can ask about the past, as they might enjoy telling you stories from long ago, as their long-term memory is often better than the short-term memory.

Below is a link to a poem on hints of ways to give dignified care to a person with dementia.

Poem – 16 things I would want if I got dementia by Rachael Wonderlin (2014)

Rachael Wonderlin, a consultant and author, has written a poem with so many practical respectful hints of how to support someone with dementia.

Free poster of this poem – https://dementiabyday.com/product/16-things-poster/

Dementia by Day – Consultant, author & podcast host – Rachael Wonderlin – https://rachaelwonderlin.com

Embracing reality short video by Rachael – www.youtube.com/watch?app=desktop&v=WovKSfdo5u8

See also – Accepting the gift of caregiving – https://acceptingthegiftofcaregiving.com/wishes-to-remember/

3. Palliative caring

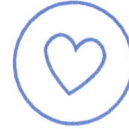

3.1 Holistic approach

Palliative care is a term used for those with dementia or any other number of medical conditions, nearing the end of their life, and needing care, more for comfort, as usually they have no hope of a cure.

Palliative care is a holistic approach, with health care professionals in the team in close communication with the patient and caregivers looking for supportive resources.

Palliative care is treatment, care and support to help people with a life-limiting illness live as comfortably as possible. When there is no curative therapy available, a palliative care team can help with symptom control, providing support and counselling, and answering questions families may have. One important aspect of palliative care is memory making, creating and capturing special moments that people can cherish forever.

Radbruch, L., Payne, S. (2009). White paper on standards and norms for hospice and palliative care in Europe: part 1. European Journal of Palliative Care, 16(6), p.278–89.

Cancer Institute NSW (2005). Turning moments into treasured memories through palliative care – www.cancer.nsw.gov.au/what-we-do/news/turning-moments-into-treasured-memories-through-pa

Depression

In Australian nursing homes, older people are increasingly frail and being admitted to care later than before. More than half of residents suffer from depression, yet psychiatrists and psychologists aren't easily accessible, and pastoral care only available for some.

Depression at the end of life is often associated with loss of meaning. Research shows people who suffer from such loss die earlier than those who maintain purpose. This can be helped by providing spiritual care that can give someone meaning and purpose.

Hopelessness

Many people have feelings of hopelessness when their physical, mental and social functions are diminished. A 95-year-old man may wonder if it's worth going on living when his wife is dead, his children don't visit and he's unable to do many things.

The suffering experienced in such situations can be understood in terms of threatening one's intactness and mourning what has been lost, including self-identity. Fear is also common among those facing death, but for different reasons. Some may be afraid of suffocating; others of ghosts, or even fear meeting their dead mother-in-law again.

What plagues people the most though, is the thought of dying alone or being abandoned (though a significant minority express a preference to die alone). Anxiety about dying usually increases after losing a loved one. But such losses can be transcended by encouraging people to pursue their own purpose for as long as they can.

Doyle, C., & Jackson, D. (2016). Spiritual care at the end of life can add purpose and help maintain identity. *The Conversation.* – https://theconversation.com/spiritual-care-at-the-end-of-life-can-add-purpose-and-help-maintain-identity-55636

3.2 Spiritual care

Spiritual care helps people care in grief, crisis and ill health, and increases their ability to recover and keep living. It also has positive impacts on behaviour and well-being.

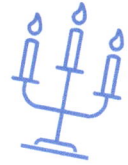

Spiritual care has religious overtones that make it an uncomfortable concept in a secular health system. But such care can be useful for all – religious and non-religious – and can be provided by carers, psychologists and pastoral specialists alike.

Spiritually can be defined as the way individuals seek and express meaning and purpose and the way they experience their connectedness to the moment, to self, to others, to nature, and to the significant or sacred". Perhaps the Japanese term *ikigai* – meaning that which gives life significance or provides a reason to get up in the morning – most closely encompasses spirituality in the context of spiritual care.

For instance, one person requested that her favourite football team regalia be placed around her room as she was dying. Another wanted her dog to stay with her in her last hours. Supporting these facets of identity can facilitate meaning and transcend the losses and anxiety associated with dying.

Some people may seek religion as they near the end of their lives, or after a traumatic event, while others who have had lifelong relationships with a church can abandon their faith at this stage.

Other components of spiritual care can include:

- Allowing people to access and recount their life story
  (see *biography therapy & dignity therapy* in second section of the handbook)

- Getting to know them, being present with them

- Understanding what is sacred to them and helping them to connect with it

- Mindfulness and meditation

- Those seeking out religious rituals, spiritual care can include reading scripture and praying.

Doyle, C., & Jackson, D. (2016). Spiritual care at the end of life can add purpose and help maintain identity. *The Conversation.* https://theconversation.com/spiritual-care-at-the-end-of-life-can-add-purpose-and-help-maintain-identity-55636

More on spiritual care:

Meaningful Aging Australia – incorporating Spiritual Health Association
https://meaningfulageing.org.au

Dementia & spiritual care short guide – https://meaningfulageing.org.au/product/dementia-and-spiritual-care-short-guide/

PART 2: Practice caring lullabies

4.   Reminiscence Therapy

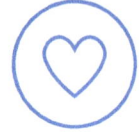

4.1   Nostalgia

Reminiscence therapy can involve thinking nostalgically about the past. Nostalgia is a bittersweet—albeit predominantly positive—self-relevant and social emotion that arises from reflecting on fond and meaningful autobiographical memories. Nostalgia might facilitate successful aging by serving as a way give emphasis to selective memories that are valuable to feel better in the face of limited time left in life.

"Now the harvest of old age is, as I have often said, the memory and rich store of blessings laid up earlier in life" – *Cicero, Cato Maior de Senectute (44 BC).*

Nostalgia as a bittersweet, but primarily positive, emotion arising from fond and personally meaningful memories that usually involve childhood or close relationships. Nostalgia often entails rose-tinted views of the memory, missing it, and a desire to return to the past; one typically feels sentimental and happy with a tinge of longing (Hepper et al., 2020).

Nostalgia has regulatory properties. Individuals spontaneously turn to personal nostalgia for comfort and strength in the face of psychological threats, and inducing it confers psychological benefits (Routledge et al., 2013). For example, experimental and cross-sectional studies show that individuals recruit and experience nostalgia in times of loneliness, discontinuity, and existential doubt. Nostalgia then repairs and enhances social connectedness, self-regard, and meaning in life (Routledge et al., 2011).

Hepper, E. G., Wildschut, T., Sedikides, C., Robertson, S., & Routledge, C. D. (2020). Time capsule: Nostalgia shields psychological wellbeing from limited time horizons. Emotion. American Psychological Association.

Walls, Y. (2021) Learning to heal, learning to dance and something accomplished: Nostalgia as social-emotional resource, a micro-study. Academic Letters, Nov 2021.

Routledge C., Arndt, J., Wildschut, T., Sedikides, C., Hart, C., Juhl, J., Vingerhoets, A. J., & Scholtz, W. (2011). The past makes the present meaningful: Nostalgia as an existential resource. Journal of Personality and Social Psychology, 101, 638-652. doi:10.1037/a0024292

Routledge, C., Wildschut, T., Sedikides, C., & Juhl, J. (2013). Nostalgia as a resource for psychological health and well-being. Social and Personality Psychology Compass, 7, p.808-818.

NOTE: Elders share stories

In older traditional cultures, it is the role of the elders to share their valued stories of old with the next generations.

See more in first section – 1. Dignity of Indigenous elderly

4.2   Reminiscence

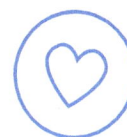

Reminiscence, that incorporates nostalgia, is the concept that recollection is an expansion of consciousness. Individual reminiscence therapy can be used in the home care setting to promote health for elderly.

Ellis, M L. (1994). Reminiscence therapy: A nursing intervention in the home care setting. Journal of Home Health Care Practice, 6(3), p. 45-51.

Reminiscence therapy involves conversations about an older person's past events and experiences. It is often done using photos and videos.

Groups of older people have become more vocal and more visible in their struggle to improve their lives. The most effective efforts to improve their situation will involve a reconceptualization of aging in a more positive light. In much of the literature the concept of reminiscence has been oversimplified and treated within a framework that views aging as decline and deterioration. Yet reminiscence the process or practice of thinking or telling about past experiences-is descriptive of a complex environment interaction which is vital to both the old and the young. It also facilitates a more positive view of aging.

Beaton, S.R. (1980), Reminiscence in old age. Nursing Forum, 19, p. 270-283.

Reminiscence therapy is a form of talk therapy. It was originally developed for use with people living with dementia but is also being used to reduce experiences of social isolation in older adults. It is defined as the process of thinking about or telling someone or a group of people about past experiences that are personally significant.

Exercising memory in this way is thought to stimulate mental activity while boosting positive feelings to create a sense of wellbeing. Reminiscence therapy can be conducted using photos, videos, or any objects from a particular period that might serve as tangible prompts to trigger nostalgic memories.

There are three categories of reminiscence therapy, namely:
- **Simple reminiscence** – Simple reminiscence is the recall and sharing of selected personal and shared memories and stories. It is mainly unstructured.
- **Life review** – Life review is a structured approach and is usually conducted individually, covering the whole life story chronologically. It aims to integrate negative and positive memories.
- **Life review therapy** – Life review therapy is a more systematic approach, typically aimed at people with depression or other mental health difficulties where the aim is to re-evaluate negative memories, promoting a more positive view of life.

Group therapy – When performed as a group, reminiscence therapy can foster friendships and a sense of belonging. Group reminiscence therapy appears to be effective in improving life satisfaction and decreasing the loneliness of people in residential aged care.

Aged Care Research & Industry Innovation. (2025). Reminiscence Therapy – www.ariia.org.au/knowledge-implementation-hub/social-isolation/social-isolation-evidence-themes/reminiscence-therapy
Care Side. (2025) Reminiscence therapy for dementia patients – www.thecareside.com.au/resources/reminiscence-therapy-for-dementia/
Wholihan D. (1992). The value of reminiscence in hospice care. *American Journal of Hospice and Palliative Medicine*, 9(2), p. 33-35.

5.   Music Therapy

Music therapy can help with reminiscence of nostalgic memories, especially with older people who have a life-time of memories that are often connected with music.

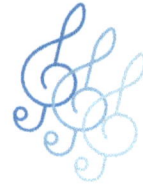

5.1   What is music therapy

Music therapy, as a profession, originated in the 1950s to help relieve the physical and emotional trauma experienced by war veterans. The demand for trained professionals steadily grew and, as a result, the Australian Music Therapy Association (AMTA) was established in 1975.

AMTA defines music therapy as "a research-based practice and profession in which music is used to actively support people as they strive to improve their health, functioning and wellbeing".

Music therapy is beneficial for people with a wide range of health concerns, including people with dementia and brain injuries.

It is a diverse practice encompassing a variety of techniques but it is based on two fundamental methods. The receptive method involves music listening, while the active method focuses on playing instruments.

Qualified music therapists work with people of any age and ability, culture and background. They will set out specific objectives and implement a tailored plan to help the individual achieve their goals. Common goals in music therapy include the development of:

- Communication skills – using vocal/verbal sounds and gestures
- Social skills – making eye contact, turn-taking, initiating interaction, and self-esteem
- Sensory skills – through touch, music listening, and levels of awareness
- Physical skills – fine and gross motor control and movement
- Cognitive skills – concentration and attention, imitation, and sequencing
- Emotional skills – expression of feelings non-verbally

IRT is one of Australia's largest community-based seniors lifestyle and care providers.

IRT *'originally known as Illawarra Retirement Trust'* was founded by Dr Max Diment and a group of likeminded people in 1969. Dr Diment had a vision; to provide seniors with better options in housing and care. This vision was inspired by Dr Diment's role as Medical Superintendent at Bulli Hospital in NSW.

IRT – community seniors lifestyle & providers –
www.irt.org.au/the-good-life/music-therapy-in-aged-care/

See also: Music therapy for seniors video
www.youtube.com/watch?v=Xx3gfEDD1z0

5.2   Benefits of music therapy in aged care

Music therapy has proven to be highly effective for older adults, especially in aged care settings. It enhances mental health, can lift mood, reduce anxiety, encourage movement, and even help manage pain.

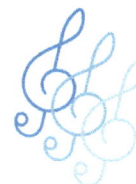

Music taps into deep emotional and sensory pathways, making it especially powerful for older adults. It can bring back special memories, provide comfort and create a sense of belonging. Whether it's a toe-tapping classic from the 50s or a calming instrumental, music has the ability to soothe, energise or simply help someone feel more connected, both to themselves and those around them.

There are many proven physical and emotional benefits and advantages of music therapy, including:

1. **Reduced anxiety** and physical effects of stress: Music has the ability to relive emotional and physical health stress, especially when combined with movement or stimulation of different sensory paths.

2. Positive impact on **healing and recovery:** It's suggested that music can positively alter the release of stress hormones that help neurological, immune and respiratory function involved in healing.

3. Management of Alzheimer's disease and **dementia**: Studies have shown that music therapy interventions can have a positive effect on motor improvement, control of emotional functions, improvements in daily activities and overall improved quality of life.

4. **Reduced depression** and other symptoms in older people: Along with physical health benefits for older people, music therapy can improve social, psychological, intellectual and cognitive performance. Both active and passive music therapy methods can improve mood and provide a sense of relief for caregivers.

5. **Improved self-expression** and communications: For those with mental health condition or physical disabilities, music therapy can help stimulate responses and improve verbal and non-verbal responses.

IRT – community seniors lifestyle & providers –
www.irt.org.au/the-good-life/music-therapy-in-aged-care/

Music connection for dementia

For people living with dementia, music can spark moments of joy, connection, and recognition, even when other forms of communication are challenging. Familiar songs often unlock long-forgotten memories or emotions, sometimes helping a person recall names, places or experiences. Music therapy can also ease confusion or agitation, creating calm and meaningful moments, even in later stages of memory decline.

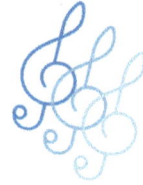

It can also have a strong influence on our mindset and emotional wellbeing. This makes the practice of clinical music therapy a great tool for relieving a range of physical and mental health conditions, including dementia.

The use of music therapy for dementia patients is a well-researched phenomenon. Dementia causes changes in cognitive functions, including decision making, judgement, memory, special orientations, reasoning and verbal communication. Dementia is also linked to behavioural and personality changes, depending on the areas affected in the brain.

By applying music therapy in aged care settings, people can experience profound benefits.

1. Awakens parts of the brain to improve mood

In people living with dementia, music therapy can awaken parts of the brain that are not impacted by dementia. It can evoke responses such as singing or humming and even moments of reconnection with loved ones. This can help reduce acute or chronic pain, ease agitation and support emotional well being.

Professor Felicity Baker, the Head of Music Therapy at the University of Melbourne, uses singing and songwriting to ease the behavioural and emotional symptoms of dementia.

"When you hear a piece of music and then the memories become evoked as a result of that, the neural network is activated, and it also then leads to the activation of more positive moods," she says. *"One of the beautiful things about music is that it takes participants in an agitated state back to safe and pleasurable memories, helping to bring them out of their shells."*

IRT – community seniors lifestyle & providers
– www.irt.org.au/the-good-life/music-therapy-in-aged-care/

28

2. Helps with memory and language

Prof Baker says older people tend to remember, and have the most connection with, music from their late teens and early 20s. *"The music stimulates those memories and with those memories comes language. If they're in early-stage dementia, and more cognitively able, we might start with dialogue around their life and connection with music."*

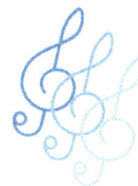

In a 10-week pilot study in Melbourne in 2017, Prof Baker's team monitored the benefits of music therapy for a group of aged care residents living with dementia. She found the progress of implementing music therapy in aged care can be marked. *"Participants are calmer, better-engaged with other people, and seemingly happier,"* she said at the time.

Prof Baker is now leading an international study on the effects of home-based music interventions on people living with dementia. Training of family carers to use music interventions in the home is being used in Australia, the United Kingdom, Norway, Poland and Germany to use music interventions to manage behavioural and psychological symptoms of dementia.

"What we want to do is observe how the use of music positively transforms their behaviour and enables them to connect more with their family members, and creates a less stressful environment," Prof Baker said.

3. Improves dementia symptoms

Another study, from the Anglia Ruskin University in Cambridge, found residents with dementia who underwent music therapy saw improvements to their symptoms.

The study took place in two care homes, both with a music therapy group and control group who did not participate in music therapy. All groups consisted of residents who had some form of dementia.

In addition to standard care, participants in the intervention group received 1:1 music therapy once a week, over a period of five months. The group showed improvements in their dementia symptoms and wellbeing, as well as a decline in disruptiveness to staff.

IRT – community seniors lifestyle & providers
– www.irt.org.au/the-good-life/music-therapy-in-aged-care/

5.3   Music therapy methods

The best music for therapy is often the most personal. Therapists work with individuals and families to choose songs that are familiar and meaningful, whether that's a childhood lullaby, a favourite hymn or music from their early adult years.

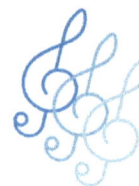

Gentle classical music, calming music, nature sounds and rhythm-based activities like drumming are also commonly used. The key is to match the music to the person's mood, preferences and needs in the moment. Because it's tailored to each person's preferences and needs, the effectiveness of music therapy is higher and offers a gentle, engaging way to support wellbeing.

Music is an integral part of daily life. Turning on the radio while driving, listening to music while cooking or creating a playlist to motivate ourselves during exercise is second nature for many of us. Music plays a fundamental role in our identity, culture and heritage and can evoke powerful memories and emotions.

Music therapy can play an important role in the care of older people, with many of the 400+ qualified music therapists in Australia working in aged care settings.

Music therapy can help seniors and people living with dementia express their feelings, communicate with others and prompt memories through music listening, singing, song writing or playing instruments.

Common music therapy methods include:

- Playing live or recorded music

- Facilitating song choice

- Active music making and improvisation

- *'Musical life review'* where the person and/or their loved ones make a compilation of music that is meaningful to them.

There is also a special technique that is used by therapists in which music is improvised to match and slow a person's breathing rate to help reduce the need for medication.

IRT – community seniors lifestyle & providers
– www.irt.org.au/the-good-life/music-therapy-in-aged-care/

More music therapy:

Music therapy – Medical & Aged Care Group
– www.maacg.com.au/residential-aged-care/music-therapy

Music intervention with older adults (Chinese) – Ma, G., Ma., X. (2023). Music intervention for older adults: Evidence map of systematic reviews. *Medicine (Baltimore)*. 2023 Dec 1;102(48):e36016. – https://pmc.ncbi.nlm.nih.gov/articles/PMC10695625/

5.4 Sing of dignity – Music for elderly

You'll never walk alone

When you walk through a storm
Hold your head up high
And don't be afraid of the dark
At the end of the storm
Is a golden sky
And the sweet silver
song of a lark

Walk on through the wind
Walk on through the rain
Tho' your dreams be
tossed and blown
Walk on, walk on
With hope in your heart
And you'll never walk alone
You'll never walk alone
Oscar Hammerstein (1945)

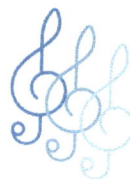

You'll never walk alone –
lyrics Oscar Hammerstein, music Richard Rodgers, for musical Carousel, 1945.

This song is a favourite song for so many special occasions of celebration and for hope during dark times, from football teams internationally as their anthem, to therapeutic sing-a-longs with elderly suffering dementia.

Sing Along for Seniors, Dementia, Memory Care, Alzheimer's

Sing-a-longs can be enjoyable for the seniors in nursing homes, retirement communities, dementia care, memory care, assisted living, and adult day programs.

One example that can be accessed online is: Sing Along with Susie Q. This website has access to hundreds of sing-along video playlists. Here is one of the songs:

You'll Never Walk Alone sing-along with on-screen lyrics
Susie Q, Praise & Joy – www.singalongwithsusieq.com
– www.youtube.com/watch?v=up7Ik038doQ

A couple of other popular songs on You Tube:
*Sentimental Journey
– www.youtube.com/watch?v=BgbiarGWJk4&list=RDBgbiarGWJk4&start_radio=1

*Unchained melody
– www.youtube.com/watch?v=AUkYES06gW4&list=RDAUkYES06gW4&start_radio=1
Aged Care Music Resources – https://agedcaremusicresources.com
See more songs next page

Songs for dignity and comfort in end-of-life care

Just a few choice songs to feel supported and loved, with links to videos with lyrics.

Abide with me – by Henry Francis Lyte (1847)*
 – www.youtube.com/watch?v=xRHUebvPsig

Amazing grace – by John Newton (1779)*
 – www.youtube.com/watch?v=HHx05uZHj1I

At your side – the Corrs (2000)
 – www.youtube.com/watch?v=bwB9EMpW8eY

Be not afraid – by Bob Dufford (1975)*
 – www.youtube.com/watch?v=kOHua5B_nqc

Bridge over troubled waters – by Simon & Garfunkel (1970)
 – www.youtube.com/watch?v=h0n-mYqB9WQ

Compassion (Change the world) – by Andrew Witt (2009)
 – www.youtube.com/watch?v=bwB9EMpW8eY

Count on me – by Bruno Mars (2010)
 – www.youtube.com/watch?v=R533DDds3RY

Don't give up – by Peter Gabriel (1986)
 – www.youtube.com/watch?v=bwB9EMpW8eY

Everybody hurts – R.E.M. (1992)
 – www.youtube.com/watch?v=FfggUztyO00

Gracias a la vida – Thank you for life – by Chilian Violeta Parra (1966)
 – sung by Mercedes Sosa (Spanish & English) – www.youtube.com/watch?v=jAlKfFLFnRI

I won't let go – by Steve Robson and Jason Sellers, sung by Rachel Flatts (2010)
 – www.youtube.com/watch?v=NX7SSAkA1Lw

Lean on me when you're not strong – Gospel song by Bill Withers (1972)
 – www.youtube.com/watch?v=iouTzcAiAR

Let me be there in your morning – by John Rostill, sung by Oliver Newton-John
 – www.youtube.com/watch?v=bwB9EMpW8eY

Stand by you – by Rachel Platten (2015)
 – www.youtube.com/watch?v=bwB9EMpW8eY

The Lord's my shepherd – by Francis Rous (1650) based on Psalm 23*
 – www.youtube.com/watch?v=9zeMcdh26YA

Try a little kindness – by Curt Sapaugh & Bobby Austin – sung by Glenn Campbell
 – www.youtube.com/watch?v=NIsGkTuO1vk

You are my sunshine – by Jimmie Davis & Charles Mitchell (1939)
 – www.youtube.com/watch?v=a5cllgM46gs

You'll never walk alone – by Oscar Hammerstein & Richard Rogers (1945)
 – www.youtube.com/watch?v=kOHua5B_nqc

You're got a friend by Carole King (1971)
 – www.youtube.com/watch?v=BcJbzuyp6VY

What a friend we have in Jesus – by Joseph M Scrivin (1855) to comfort his mother*
 – www.youtube.com/watch?v=TAyaXdvvbGU

* Christian specific words of comfort

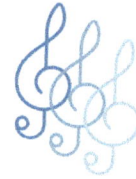

32

6. *Song of Life* biographical music therapy

Song of Life (SOL) intervention is a biographical music therapy for end-of-life palliative care.

Patients nearing the end-of-life report high needs for emotional and spiritual support. Although the use of psychosocial interventions including life review and creative arts-based techniques is immensely valued in clinical practice, recent guidelines, reviews, and reports have repeatedly called for high-quality studies on their efficacy.

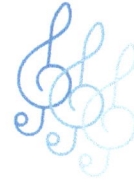

Findings show that biographical music therapy can effectively facilitate psycho-spiritual integration of past life events. The intervention was further effective in reducing patients' momentary distress and was perceived as meaningful and important by both patients and family members.

The *Song of Life* (SOL) intervention was provided on two consecutive sessions containing:

1. Biographical interview to determine a biographical meaningful song

2. A live performance of a song with biographical relevance to the patient as a lullaby

6.1 Biographical interview

The first session comprises an interview including biographical questions with a focus on the musical background of the person. The aim is to identify the patient's *song of life*, which is a song that has a high biographical relevance and the potential to arouse strong emotional reactions. Such a song is often associated with social bounds (e.g. romantic partner, children, parents), biographic events (e.g. marriage, child's birth), or certain places (e.g. birthplace, vacation). The first session ends with the offer to perform a brief music therapy relaxation exercise using the monochord and vocal improvisation.

6.2 Meaningful biographical song performance

The second session, next day, is to give the therapist time to prepare the patient's song of life. The therapist uses the guitar/piano and her voice and first initiates a brief relaxation exercise accompanied by gentle sounds on the instrument in the musical key of the following song. The therapist gradually reduces the meter. If applicable, the therapist can include quotations of important sentences from the interview in the song. The music afterwards turns into a life performance of the SOL in a lullaby style. This recorded and played back to the patient, followed by a conversation about themes and feedback, and then playing the song again.

Warth, M., Kessler, J., van Kampen, J., Ditzen, B., Bardenheuer, H. J. (2018).'Song of Life': music therapy in terminally ill patients with cancer. British Medical Journal Support Palliative Care. Jun 2018;8(2), p.167-170. – https://pubmed.ncbi.nlm.nih.gov/29500238/

Warth, M., Koehler, F., Weber, M., Bardenheuer, H.J., Ditzen, B., Kessler, J. (2019). "Song of Life (SOL)" study protocol: a multicenter, randomized trial on the emotional, spiritual, and psychobiological effects of music therapy in palliative care. British Medical Centre Palliative Care. Jan 2019, 30;18(1):14. – https://pubmed.ncbi.nlm.nih.gov/30700278/

7. Biography Therapy

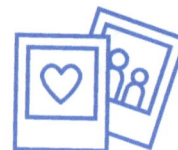

Dr Ivan Litcher, was head of the Te Omaga hospice program in New Zealand in the early 90s, and noticed that many approaching the end of life appeared to feel hopeless and depressed, believing their lives had no meaning. So he came up with a biography program, wanting the patients to feel valued, and have a more peaceful end in life.

Storytelling has always been a universal powerful tool used to maintain one's sense meaning in life, one's heritage, to hand over important traditions and rituals and to convey lessons to be learnt. It is a means of passing on what matters.

A number of people in palliative care choose to revisit painful memories or share secrets with their biographers that they never want recorded in the story. Comments such as *'I don't want this written in, but I just needed to tell someone',* are commonplace. There is safety for our clients in engaging in honest conversation with their biographers and all of this can contribute to a more peaceful death on behalf of the client.

Rice, M. (2022, June 29). Biography service for the dying: A legacy and therapy. Good Grief! https://good-grief.com.au/biography-service-for-the-dying-a-legacy-and-therapy/

7.1 Biographical story recorded

Often biography volunteers worker at palliative care facilities, like Eastern Palliative Care in Melbourne, work one on one with our clients allowing them to tell their story. Biography recording often takes place over six to ten visits of one hour in duration.

7.2 Meaningful story as legacy

The process of storytelling enables messages, philosophies, beliefs, memories and culture to pass from one person to the next.

Engaging in the process also allows the client to place the current medicalised experience of a palliative illness back into the broader context of their life – to understand their current *'care recipient'* role is not what ultimately defines them. It allows each client to reconnect with the essence of who they are and remember they are larger than their diagnosis.

Clients report a rise in a sense of wellbeing and a decrease in levels of depression, anxiety, breathlessness, and pain as a result of the biography intervention.

Eastern Palliative Care (2025) Biography – www.epcvic.org.au/biography

Hesse, M., Forstmeier, S., Cuhls, H. *et al.* (2019). Volunteers in a biography project with palliative care patients – a feasibility study. *BMC Palliative Care* 18, 79.

Creating a life story book – a form of biography therapy

A life story book is a wonderful way to bring back memories for a person living with dementia, and at the same time provide useful information to caregivers about that person.

It can be as simple or as complex as you wish to make it.

Start with photographs of the person and a description of their history.
Keep information positive, avoid tragic events or memories that may cause the person distress or emotional upheaval.

Organise the information into a photo album, scrapbook or by using an online photo book service. Include a variety of photographs from the person's past and present.

The life story could include:

- The person's full name and preferred name
- Date and place of birth, names of parents and siblings
- Description of childhood home, pets, friend's names, holidays
- Occupation, names of work colleagues
- Partner's name, how they met, date and place of wedding
- First home with partner
- Names and description of children
- Travel and holidays
- Activities and interests
- Important life events

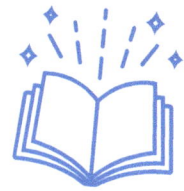

Creating a life story book – Alzheimer's WA
https://alzheimerswa.org.au/helpsheets/creating-a-life-story-book/

Creating a life story book template
– https://alzheimerswa.org.au/wp-content/uploads/2024/11/AWA-Life-Story-Template-Draft-3-003.pdf

8.   Narrative therapy for end of life

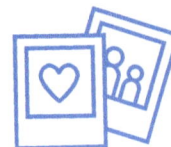

8.1   Re-membering identity

Michael White narrative therapy founder, conceived of re-membering as: evoking the image of a person's life and identity as an association or a club. The membership of this association of life is made up of the significant figures of a person's history, as well as the identities of the person's present circumstances, whose voices are influential regarding how the person constructs their own identity. (White, 2007, p. 134).

While re-membering practices are commonly used to *'support people to reposition themselves in relation to the death of a loved one, in ways that bring relief'* (White, 2007, p. 135).

8.2   Re-membering from dying mothers for their children

Tanya Newman shares stories of dying mothers writing letters for their children in her article: *"Love always": Letters written by dying mothers for their children.*
The author conceives of letter writing as a way for mothers to re-member their preferred identities, and the letters as portals for future re-membering for children. The article includes examples of questions asked in interviews with mothers, the thinking behind the questions, and excerpts from the letters these conversations enabled.

Through a mother's loving eyes

Interviews were started with questions that invited descriptions of the children. This was a way to warm up the conversation, with each woman introducing her children to me. Mothers would up as she spoke and relax into sharing their stories. The questions included:

- Could you introduce [child] to me?
- What can you tell me about [child]?
- What are some of your best memories of [child]?
- If [child] were to see themself through your eyes, what would they see?

An example of the content generated through these questions is:

> *"You are an amazing kid. You brighten up a room when you come in. It makes me proud, the way you speak up if something's not right. I appreciate how you let others know they are loved by doing kind things and saying: 'I love you'. When I think of the way we say, 'I love you', 'I love you more!', 'No, I love you more!', it makes me smile. I hope I have taught you to love easily and whole heartedly. You are kind and gentle: all the beautiful things that anyone would want in a son. And you give the best hugs. I love sinking into your hugs. They're so big and strong and real."*

Newman, T. (2025). "Love always": Letters written by dying mothers for their children. *International Journal of Narrative Therapy and Community Work*, (2), 11–20. – https://dulwichcentre.com.au/wp-content/uploads/2025/09/Newman_LoveAlwaysLettersDyingMothers_IJNTCW_20252.pdf

White, M. (2007). *Maps of narrative practice*. Norton.

9.   Dignity therapy

Dignity therapy by Dr Harvey Chochinoy of Canada

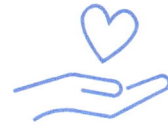

Dignity Therapy

Dignity Therapy offers patients a
safe space to explore their life's
meaning and articulate their final messages,
whether it is for their self-reflection and closure,
or as a cherished keepsake for family and friends.

9.1   Care with dignity

What do I need to know about you to give you the best care I can?

Dignity Therapy often begins with the patient dignity question (PDQ) consisting of a brief (approximately ten-minute) conversation, framed the question: *What do we need to know about you as a person to take the best care of you possible.* Patients are encouraged to provide reflections on personhood and how they would like to be known or seen by their healthcare providers. PDQ responses often include reflections pertaining to:

- Values and beliefs
- Relationships
- Worries and concerns
- Roles and responsibilities
- History and stories

Research has shown that this single question can identify issues and stressors that may be important to consider when planning and delivering someone's care and treatment. The intent is to reveal the *'invisible'* factors that might not otherwise come to light – and to identify these concerns early in the process.

9.2   Connect with dignity

Any person you want to reconnect with?

Dignity Therapy was developed by Dr. Harvey Max Chochinov to assist people dealing with the imminent end of their lives.

This brief intervention can help conserve the dying patient's sense of dignity by addressing sources of psychosocial and existential distress. It gives patients a chance to record the meaningful aspects of their lives and leave something behind that can benefit their loved ones in the future.

During a 30 to 60 minute session, the therapist asks a series of open-ended questions that encourage patients to talk about their lives or what matters most to them. The conversation is recorded, transcribed, edited and then returned within a few days to the patient, who is given the opportunity to read the transcript and make changes before a final version is produced. Many choose to share the document with family and friends.

9.2   Connect with dignity (continued)

Dignity therapy gives patients an opportunity to share the moments that shaped their lives.

Dignity therapy borrows elements from other supportive techniques, such as life review, logotherapy and existential psychotherapy. Unlike life review, dignity therapy is not a historical recounting of events – it is a recounting of thoughts, ideas and events that are particularly relevant and meaningful for patients to recount and pass along to others. For most patients, it is an opportunity to share the moments that shaped their lives.

An important difference of dignity therapy is its grounding in sound research into dying patients' self-reported notions of dignity. It addresses the dying patient's need to feel that life has had meaning, and to do something for loved ones that will endure beyond the patient's own life. It also helps the patient get in touch with the accomplishments and experiences that have made them unique and valued human beings.

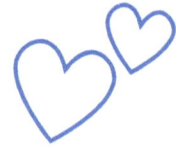

9.3   Communicate with dignity

What legacy do you want to leave?

Dignity therapy deals with emotional pain by targeting its source. The content, protocol and questions are all guided by the dignity model sub-themes.

The dying patient's strong need for *'generativity'* and *'legacy'* is the basis for the therapy. The therapy creates something that will transcend the patient's death and extend his or her influence across time. Capturing the patient's thoughts in written form is particularly effective because it increases the sense that whatever is said will be preserved for the future.

However, simply creating the legacy document is not enough. Those who practice dignity therapy must listen to these stories with genuine empathy, attentiveness, interest and sensitivity. Anything less will fail to meet the patient's need for treatment that is unconditionally positive and caring in tone.

The questions asked during dignity therapy are shaped by the dignity-conserving perspectives and aftermath concerns that are identified in the dignity model. Each area of inquiry lets patients speak to issues that may reinforce their sense of personhood and sustain a sense of meaning, purpose and self-worth – thereby decreasing distress and improving their quality of life.

Dignity in care – Dr Harvey Chochinov & team, Canada – https://dignityincare.ca/en/

Chochinov, H. M., Hack, T., Hassard, T., Kristjanson, L. J., McClement, S., & Harlos, M. (2005). Dignity Therapy: A Novel Psychotherapeutic Intervention for Patients Near the End of Life. *Journal of Clinical Oncology*, *23*(24), 5520–5525. – https://doi.org/10.1200/JCO.2005.08.391

Chochinov, H. M. (2014). *Dignity therapy: Final words for final days.* Oxford University Press.

10. Practice of dignity therapy

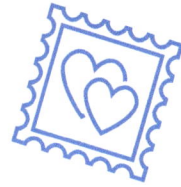

(with reminiscence & biography therapy within dignity therapy)

Seek and ye shall find.   **Knock** and the door will be open

Ask and it shall be given   When the **love** comes trickling down

Gospel song by Stephen C Foster (1863)

10.1   Seek special times

Seek out stories of special times in their lives – and ye will find – briefly document their stories to find treasures for them and their families. Plus, check for any stories of disruption with fractured relationships and offer to help write a letter for healing and to reconcile. *(Reminiscence Therapy, Biography Therapy, & Dignity Therapy).*

Ask about the sparkling moments in their lives – any special rituals or traditions or memorable one-off events – to be briefly documented, perhaps with any relevant photos they have, to be copied and added. *(Narrative Therapy & Appreciative Inquiry)*

Check if there are any fractured relationships in the family or close friends that they might like to try and reconcile if possible. This could take the form of a letter that the person in question, with an apology that they have not been in contact, and they would like to make amends and try to repair, before it is too late. Thus the relationship can have some healing.

10.2   Knock for family photos and travels

Knock and the door will be open – Knock to find out about **photos of family & friends** – as a door or window to their souls. Look at family photos around the room - make up a booklet or album of photos with names underneath, or add names to photos around room, so they remember the names for longer *(to help with dementia)*/ Open the door to **travels** - find photos or find images online that they relate too – make up a booklet of photos with short descriptions of each, to bring back happy memories and wisdom learnt by exploring their adventures in the world *(to improve self-esteem).*

A small booklet can be made with copies of photos from friends and family and/or from travels with a label underneath each, on plain paper and stapled together to have in one place. There are also many creative ways to use the photos. Here are some ideas below.

10 ways to use the power of photos with dementia memory loss
Alzheimers Texes - The state of mind – www.txalz.org/blog/powerofphotos/

How images can help dementia sufferers engage with life – Australian Psychological Society
www.psychologytoday.com/au/blog/caring-the-caregivers/202105/how-images-can-help-dementia-sufferers-engage-life

Knock to find out favourite places in **travel** or would like to travel too.

Travel with dementia – Dementia Australia
– https://www.dementia.org.au/living-dementia/staying-connected/travelling-dementia

Supported holidays for dementia – Dementia Adventures
– https://dementiaadventure.org/holidays/

10.3   Ask for favourite music, foods & nature

MUSIC

Ask and it shall be given – ask about favourite **music.** Find and play back favourite music together to cheer them. If they like to sing along print out the words in large print *(to help with dementia or catatonic state)*

Music for dementia - Forward with dementia
– https://forwardwithdementia.au/news/music-and-dementia/FOOD

Ask about favourite **food** – like chocolate, fruit or ice-cream. Bring food to share *(to boost the mood and connect)*.

Eating & Dementia - Dementia Australia
– www.dementia.org.au/living-dementia/home-life/eating-and-dementia

Brain boosting food for dementia

- Colourful fruits, berries & vegetables
- Fish
- Nuts & seeds & wholegrains

Brain boosting food for dementia
– www.uhhospitals.org/blog/articles/2023/01/5-brain-boosting-foods-that-can-fight-dementia

NOTE: Ma*ggie Beer Foundation* – Creating an appetite for life – Delivering education and training to improve the dining, food, and nutritional outcomes for older people in Aged Care. – https://maggiebeerfoundation.org.au

NATURE

Ask about places in **nature**, perhaps with favourite walks. If they are able, go for a walk in nature, or watch a documentary on nature together or a travel documentary together *(to help calm)*.

Benefits of connection with nature and outdoor activity - Dementia Adventure
– https://dementiaadventure.org/resources/the-benefits-of-nature/

Time in nature for dementia - Hovi Care Elderly care in Bali & Singapore
– https://hovicare.com/can-spending-time-in-nature-help-manage-symptoms-of-dementia/

Green spaces, dementia and a meaningful life in community article
– www.sciencedirect.com/science/article/abs/pii/S1353829220300617

Exposure to nature gardens for dementia
– https://pubmed.ncbi.nlm.nih.gov/28835119/

Spending time in nature for dementia case study - Alzheimer's UK
– www.alzheimers.org.uk/get-support/publications-and-factsheets/dementia-together/spending-time-nature-dementia-wellbeing

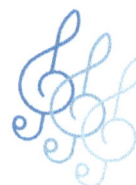

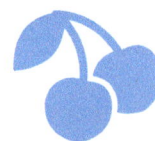

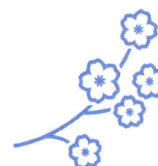

10.4   Love given to others

When the LOVE comes trickling down - feel their love of life again - remembering what they **gave to others** – to their family, friends, church or other local community group. Also, love of creative activities they have done for or with others, like sharing: stories, photos, travels, music, food and nature *(to help with dignity)*.

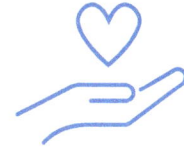

People are often grateful for what they have been given in life, especially the care they have been given towards the end of their lives.

However, these elderly people often have given much to others throughout their lives, before they became frail and needing care themselves.

So it can be good to ask about the love and care they have given to others over the years, and what legacy they are leaving for others.

They may have given much to:

- Intimate partners – compassion and care
- Children and grand-children – helping to grow and fly
- Close family and friends – supporting each others
- Colleagues – leadership and/or team work
- Neighbours – welcoming and helping
- Community group members – faith, sport, gardens, choir, art groups
- Hospitality to family and friends
- Welcoming the stranger – foster care, neighbours, migrants
- Caring for the sick - nursing
- Teaching children or adults – schools or online
- Volunteering – visitation, op shop, creating or repairing for others
- Building or mending things – in and around the home
- Creating books, music or art works – for relaxation or to publish or promote
- Providing or listening to music – composing, leading singing, playing in orchestra

Ask 'what legacy are you leaving for others?'

11. Death doula

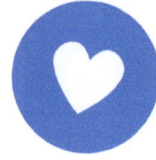

When facing death, it can be so helpful to have an experienced guide for support. Death doulas, like doulas for the birthing process, offer support

Death Doula

A death doula or death midwife or is a person who assists in the dying process, much like a midwife or doula does with the birthing process. It is often a community-based role, aiming to help families cope with death, recognising it as a natural and important part of life. The role can supplement and go beyond hospice.

during this time towards the ending of a life.

Go Gentle Australia

The word doula means 'to serve'.

There are various ways to describe a death doula, including:

- End-of-life consultant
- Death walker
- Death midwife
- Death guide

A death doula is there to serve people at the end of their lives. They enter the space with no judgement. They know the people they serve are experts in their own lives. They might sit with you, listen to you, and hold space for you to explore death and all the feelings and needs that come with it.

Doulas are a vessel of information. They don't take the place of the family, or anything medical. They are a non-medical accompaniment to health care or hospice care. They are the one constant - even after the person has died.

There are various reasons why people might want a death doula, perhaps:

- Nobody else wants to talk frankly about the end of life with you

- Worried about upsetting loved ones.

- Anxieties and would appreciate support in planning ahead
  and working out what you want, with gentle compassionate conversations

Go Gentle Australia – www.gogentleaustralia.org.au/what_is_a_death_doula

You can connect with death doulas in your state:
End of Life Doula directory – www.endoflifedouladirectory.com.au/

End of Life Doula course

Just like birth doulas support the beginning of life, death doulas support the end of life. This is a journey for both the person dying and their family, and a death doula provides the help needed to navigate this final path.

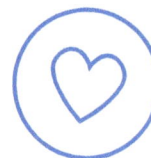

A death doula provides emotional, spiritual and physical support and works in conjunction with other services such as hospice and medical professionals. Having someone to lean on during a part of our lives that is still fairly unknown is a hugely valuable resource.

An Online End of life Doula course with Learning Cloud, is 100 hours, and can be completed online or by correspondence.

Modules include:

1. Becoming a compassionate presence
2. Companioning the dying
3. End of life choices
4. Doula skills and scope of practice
5. Expanding your skill set
6. Self-sustainability
7. Planning for care
8. Building a practice

The Peaceful Presence End of Life Doulas course
– https://thepeacefulpresenceproject.org

Enrol for End of Life Doula course at Learning Cloud (Australia)
– https://learningcloud.com.au/courses/2757/end-of-life-doula?gad_source=1&gad_campaignid=21202043729&gbraid=0AAAAADKBzZnbfpi6QX3c aZSCb39SF_sHt

Dying to know: Bringing death to life – book

Dying to Know book, aims to cut through the taboos and place death firmly in the circle of life. Quirky without being too irreverent, accessible without being glib, and challenging without being disturbing, this book is a collection of conversation starters that lifts the lid on death and helps connect us all a little more. Subjects covered include planning a personalised funeral; ways to help people who are terminally ill; making an emotional will; organ donation; creating online memorials; opening the conversation with children; things to do before you die; and much more.

Anastasios, A. (2007). *Dying to know: Bringing death to life.* Hardie Grant.

12. Dealing with grief after death

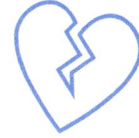

12.1   Grief Australia

Grief is a natural response to loss, with strong emotional responses towards the end of life, and by the carers of the one at the end of life. Grief can be thought of as all the love you have, but with no-where to go.

Grief is not only about loss—it often reshapes how we see ourselves. It's common for people to turn their pain inward when dealing with loss. This can lead to the bereaved treating themselves with less kindness than usual which may manifest into several responses.

Self-blame and guilt — Sometimes people torment themselves with thoughts of what they could have done differently. This could be related to things they could have done to prevent the death, or for past actions and harsh words directed the person while they were here. *'If only…'*, *'I should have…'* are common thoughts.

Harsh self-judgement — People deal with their grief in a myriad of ways and although our grief changes over time we never *'get over it'*. However, it's common for people to feel they're grieving the wrong way, or that they are taking too long to *'get over it'*. They may also criticise themselves if they catch themselves smiling or laughing after the loss of someone, feeling that it's inappropriate to experience feelings of happiness.

Neglecting self-care — Self-care rituals can often be put on the back-burner during grief, with proper nutrition, sleep and exercise being often overlooked. This could be a result of intense sadness and low energy making it difficult to take care of oneself, or feelings of *'what's the point' 'life has no meaning'*.

Isolation — Social connection is important for anyone, but particularly for those grieving loss. However, it's common for people to withdraw from social support believing they should handle their grief privately, not wanting to be a burden or bring others down.

Unrealistic expectations — People who have unrealistic expectations of the grief process and how they should handle things often set impossibly high standards for coping. If they fail to reach these standards, they can feel inadequate or a failure.

Why kindness is key

Self-kindness after loss is not an indulgence. It's a vital part of healing and working through grief. One study showed that higher levels of self-compassion were associated with lower levels of complicated grief, depression and post-traumatic stress. Another study showed that self-compassion was linked to greater resilience and post-traumatic growth among people who suffered loss.

Treating yourself with kindness and self-compassion can also help you deal with and navigate difficult or uncomfortable emotions without suppressing or exaggerating them. This balance is crucial to process grief in a healthy way.

Grief Australia – www.grief.org.au

12.2   How to navigate grief with kindness and self-compassion

While there are no rules around how to journey through grief, there are some things you can do to support yourself during this difficult time.

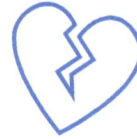

Accept that grief is normal — It's important to remember that grief is a normal part of loving someone and losing them. Acknowledging this and how you feel can gently validate your experience.

Acknowledge your pain — Acknowledge your pain and loss without judgement. This will help validate your feelings and help you grieve without feeling that the process needs to be hidden or kept from others.

Understand that healing takes time — There is no set timeline for grief, nor one way to 'do' grief. Understanding this gives you the freedom to allow for days when you feel sad, even if it's sometime after the death. It also allows for the ebbs and flow of emotions that can occur.

Be prepared for all kinds of emotions — You will experience many emotions as you grieve. These may include sadness, anger, rage, guilt, overwhelm, and helplessness. You'll also have times when you'll feel happy, despite your loss, or notice that you are looking forward to things in the future. All feelings are normal and okay to have.

Be your own best friend — Treat yourself as you would a dear friend who is going through loss. Offer yourself the same words of comfort and give yourself the permission and space to feel what you feel.

Take some time out — Take a step back from your usual responsibilities; whether it's work, study or volunteering so you have space and time to grieve and take care of yourself. Relieving the pressure of having to keep up with regular activities will help you navigate your loss.

Take care of yourself physically — Try to prioritise sleep, eating well and gentle exercise. Supporting your body physically will help you move through the grief process with more resilience and balance.

Ask for support — Reach out to family, friends or work colleagues and ask them to support you. This could be in practical ways such as picking kids up from school, taking on some of your workload, or just being available to provide emotional support when you need it. If you're struggling to cope, don't hesitate to consult a grief counsellor or therapist who can provide professional support.

Grief Australia – www.grief.org.au

Life, death & spirituality conversations audio – Meaningful Aging Australia
– https://meaningfulageing.org.au/product/how-we-are-changed-conversations-on-grief-loss-trauma-conversation-1-life-death-spirituality/

Anticipatory grief conversations audio – Meaningful Aging Australia
– https://meaningfulageing.org.au/product/how-we-are-changed-conversations-on-grief-loss-trauma-conversation-2-anticipatory-grief/

12.3   Take time to remember the person who has died

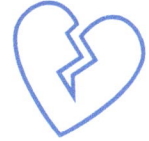

Honouring the life of the person with gentle rituals can be an act of self-compassion and connection. While they may not be physically here, they can live on in your memories and in your heart. Developing rituals and other ways to remember them can provide a sense of connection, comfort and purpose, and be an important and meaningful way to support your grief journey. Some suggestions include:

Create a memory box — Collect personal mementos such as photos, letters, cards, jewellery or any other items that have special significance and place them in a special box that you can revisit when you need to.

Plant a tree or garden — Plant a tree in their memory or turn part of your garden into a space where you can sit and remember them. You could include their favourite plants or flowers and include items that have special meaning.

Get creative — If you're creative you could write a poem, paint a picture, design a memorial quilt or create a weaving that incorporates some of their clothing.

Create a playlist — Put together a playlist of their favourite songs, or songs that you shared together and don't be afraid to include songs that put a smile on your face.

Write your stories — If you have lots of happy or funny memories, you can write them all down. You don't need to be good at writing. Just recording these moments can help you feel more connected to them and offer an opportunity to share their stories with others who knew them.

Develop new rituals — Develop new rituals to celebrate significant days. For example, celebrate their birthday with coffee and special cake, or do something to mark the anniversary of their death. You can also incorporate new rituals into occasions such as Christmas, Easter, Mother's Day and Father's Day.

Get involved in charity — Choose a charity that aligned with the person who has died, or your experience of loss and get involved. It could be by donating in their name, attending charity fun runs, or raising awareness of an important issue.

By treating yourself with gentleness and understanding, you create a supportive internal environment that will help you heal. Remember, the journey through grief is deeply personal, and is different for everyone. Be patient with yourself, honour your feelings, and allow kindness to be your companion as you move through this challenging time.

Grief is not something to *'get over'*, but something we learn to carry with kindness. As you walk this path, may you offer yourself the same grace and love you would give to a dear friend.

Specialised grief counselling and support services are available through the Grief Australia website or by calling 1800 642 066.

Grief Australia – www.grief.org.au

NOTE: **Support services**

There are many support services for the time towards the end of life, and for the carers and for those suffering from grief, both the elderly and the carers. This handbook has some support resources listed on the next pages, for some guidance.

Resources & supports

Websites

Aged Care Music Resources – https://agedcaremusicresources.com

Aged Care Quality – Australian Government – *Yarning about aged care and your rights* – www.agedcarequality.gov.au/sites/default/files/media/yarning-about-aged-care-and-your-rights-conversation-guide.pdf

Aging Mind Initiative – The University of Queensland
– https://ami.group.uq.edu.au/story-promote-empathy-dementia-care

Alzheimer's Texas – *Photos with dementia memory loss* – www.txalz.org/blog/powerofphotos/

Alzheimer's UK – *Spending time in nature for dementia case study*
– www.alzheimers.org.uk/get-support/publications-and-factsheets/dementia-together/spending-time-nature-dementia-wellbeing

Alzheimer's WA – *Creating a life story book* – https://alzheimerswa.org.au/helpsheets/creating-a-life-story-book/

Barwon Health – *Palliative care service leaves memories of great dignity*
– www.barwonhealth.org.au/news/palliative-care-service-leaves-memories-of-great-dignity/

Dementia Adventure – *Benefits of connection with nature and outdoor activity* –
– https://dementiaadventure.org/resources/the-benefits-of-nature/

Dementia Adventures – *Supported holidays for dementia* – https://dementiaadventure.org/holidays/

Dementia Australia *Travel with dementia* – www.dementia.org.au/living-dementia/staying-connected/travelling-dementia

Dementia Support Australia – *The carer handbook for understanding changed behaviours*
– www.dementia.com.au.

Dignity in Care, Canada – *Kindness, humanity & respect* – https://dignityincare.ca/en/

Eastern Palliative Care – with *biography therapy* – https://www.epcvic.org.au

End of Life Doula directory – www.endoflifedouladirectory.com.au/

Exposure to nature gardens for dementia – https://pubmed.ncbi.nlm.nih.gov/28835119/

Go Gentle Australia – *Death doulas & resources*
– www.gogentleaustralia.org.au/what_is_a_death_doula

Grief Australia – www.grief.org.au

Hovi Care Elderly care in Bali & Singapore – *Time in nature for dementia*
– https://hovicare.com/can-spending-time-in-nature-help-manage-symptoms-of-dementia/

IRT – Community seniors' lifestyle – www.irt.org.au/the-good-life/music-therapy-in-aged-care/

Jan Pentland Foundation – www.janpentlandfoundation.org

Learning Cloud – *End of life doula course* – https://thepeacefulpresenceproject.org/ & *Peaceful Presence End of Life Doulas* course – https://thepeacefulpresenceproject.org

Meaningful Aging Australia – https://meaningfulageing.org.au

Medical & Aged Care Group – www.maacg.com.au

Music Therapy for the elderly – IRS – www.irt.org.au/the-good-life/music-therapy-in-aged-care/

Music therapy – Medical & Aged Care – www.maacg.com.au/residential-aged-care/music-therapy

National Library of Medicine – *Music intervention with older adults* (Chinese)
– https://pmc.ncbi.nlm.nih.gov/articles/PMC10695625/

Palliative Care Australia – https://palliativecare.org.au

Palliative Care NSW – *Dignity therapy: Learning to create a life document*
– https://palliativecarensw.org.au/dignity-therapy/

Photos with dementia memory loss – Alzheimer's Texas – www.txalz.org/blog/powerofphotos/

Science Direct – *Green spaces, dementia and a meaningful life in community article*
– www.sciencedirect.com/science/article/abs/pii/S1353829220300617

Susie Q, Praise & Joy – www.singalongwithsusieq.com

World Health Organisation – *Palliative Care* – www.who.int/news-room/fact-sheets/detail/palliative-care

Articles and books

Aged Care Research & Industry Innovation. (2025). *Reminiscence Therapy*. Website: www.ariia.org.au/knowledge-implementation-hub/social-isolation/social-isolation-evidence-themes/reminiscence-therapy

Anastasios, A. (2007). *Dying to know: Bringing death to life*. Hardie Grant.

Bentley, B., O'Connor, M., Williams, A., Breen, L.J. (2020). Dignity therapy online: Piloting an online psychosocial intervention for people with terminal illness. *Digital Health, 2020*, Sep 20;6

Brooks, C., Sunkel, C., & Stewart, H. L. N. (2025). Dignity in mental healthcare: Service user perspectives. *Academia Mental Health and Well-Being*, 2(1). Website – www.academia.edu/2997-9196/2/1/10.20935/MHealthWellB7523#B6-sustainability-3411931

Chochinov, H. M., Hack, T., Hassard, T., Kristjanson, L. J., McClement, S., & Harlos, M. (2005). Dignity Therapy: A Novel Psychotherapeutic Intervention for Patients Near the End of Life. *Journal of Clinical Oncology*, *23*(24), 5520–5525. https://doi.org/10.1200/JCO.2005.08.391

Chochinov, H. M. (2014). *Dignity therapy: Final words for final days*. Oxford University Press.

Dementia Support Australia. (2025). *The carer handbook for understanding changed behaviours*. Website – www.dementia.com.au.

Dignity in Care. (2022). *Dignity therapy at end of life* with video – https://dignityincare.ca/en/dignity-therapy-at-end-of-life.html

Doyle, C., & Jackson, D. (2016). Spiritual care at the end of fife can add purpose and help maintain identity. *The Conversation*. https://theconversation.com/spiritual-care-at-the-end-of-life-can-add-purpose-and-help-maintain-identity-55636

Ent, M. R., & Gergis, M. A. (2020). The Most Common End-of-Life Reflections: A Survey of Hospice and Palliative Nurses. *Death Studies*, *44*(4), 256–260.

Genove, L. (2007). *Still Alice*. iUniverse. [*Still Alice* movie version – www.youtube.com/watch?v=KtZpkG36_M4]

Hanna, F. (2025). For migrants, dementia can mean losing a language and a whole world. *The Conversation*. 12 September 2025. https://theconversation.com/for-migrants-dementia-can-mean-losing-a-language-and-a-whole-world-263185

Harris, G. W. (2020). *Dignity and vulnerability: Strength and quality of character*. University of California Press.

Hesse, M., Forstmeier, S., Cuhls, H. *et al.* (2019). Volunteers in a biography project with palliative care patients – a feasibility study. *BMC Palliative Care* 18, 79.

Hughes, B. (2012). End-of-Life Chaplaincy Care. In S. Roberts (Ed.), *Professional Spiritual & Pastoral Care: A Practical Clergy and Chaplain's Handbook* (pp. 162–177). SkyLight Paths Pub.

Jenkins. (2002). Offering Spiritual Care. In B. D. Rumbold (Ed.), *Spirituality and Palliative Care: Social and Pastoral Perspectives* (pp. 116–129). Oxford University Press.

Articles and Books (continued)

Kellehear, A. (1999). *Health Promoting Palliative Care*. Oxford University Press.

Lim Y. (2023) Dignity and dignity therapy in end-of-life Care. *Journal of Hospice and Palliative Care, 2023*, 26, p.145-148. Website: www.e-jhpc.org/journal/view.html?uid=526&vmd=Full

Lothian, K., Philp, I. (2001). Maintaining the dignity and autonomy of older people in the healthcare setting. *British Medical Journal.* 17 March 2001, 322(7287), p. 668-70.

McClellan, F. M. (2020). *Healthcare and human dignity: Law matters*. Rutgers University Press.

Music therapy with Chinese elderly – Ma, G., Ma., X. (2023). Music intervention for older adults: Evidence map of systematic reviews. *Medicine (Baltimore).* 2023 Dec 1;102(48):e36016.

Newman, T. (2025). "Love always": Letters written by dying mothers for their children. *International Journal of Narrative Therapy and Community Work*, (2), 11–20. – https://dulwichcentre.com.au/wp-content/uploads/2025/09/Newman_LoveAlwaysLettersDyingMothers_IJNTCW_20252.pdf

Quill, T. E. (1994). *Death and dignity: Making choices and taking charge*. W.W. Norton.

Rice, M. (2022). Biography Service for the Dying: A Legacy and Therapy. *Good Grief!* https://good-grief.com.au/biography-service-for-the-dying-a-legacy-and-therapy/

Rubin, A., Parrish, D. E., & Miyawaki, C. E. (2019). Benchmarks for Evaluating Life Review and Reminiscence Therapy in Alleviating Depression among Older Adults. *Social Work, 64*(1), 61–72. https://doi.org/10.1093/sw/swy054

Vuksanovic, D., Green, H., & Morrissey, S. (2018). *Empirical foundations of dignity therapy: Comparing dignity therapy with life review for palliative care patients*. Griffith University.

Warth, M., Kessler, J., van Kampen, J., Ditzen, B., Bardenheuer, H. J. (2018).'Song of Life': music therapy in terminally ill patients with cancer. *British Medical Journal Support Palliative Care.* Jun 2018;8(2), p.167-170. https://pubmed.ncbi.nlm.nih.gov/29500238/

Warth, M., Koehler, F., Weber, M., Bardenheuer, H.J., Ditzen ,B., Kessler, J. (2019). "Song of Life (SOL)" study protocol: a multicenter, randomized trial on the emotional, spiritual, and psychobiological effects of music therapy in palliative care. *British Medical Centre Palliative Care.* Jan 2019, 30;18(1):14. https://pubmed.ncbi.nlm.nih.gov/30700278/

Warth, M., Koehler, F., Brehmen, M., Weber, M., Bardenheuer, H. J,. Ditzen, B., Kessler, J. (2021). "Song of Life": Results of a multicenter randomized trial on the effects of biographical music therapy in palliative care. *Palliative Medicine.* Jun 2021;35(6), p.1126-1136. https://pubmed.ncbi.nlm.nih.gov/33876660/

White, M. (2007). *Maps of narrative practice*. Norton.

Wiseman, H. (2016, December). Spiritual care at the end of life; How to reduce distress as we face dying. *Palliative Care Australia.* https://palliativecare.org.au/story/spiritual-care-at-the-end-of-life-how-to-reduce-distress-as-we-face-dying/

Woods B, O'Philbin L, Farrell E.M., Spector A.E., Orrell M. (2018). Reminiscence therapy for dementia. *Cochrane Database System Review.* 2018 Mar 2018, 1;3(3).

Copyright Permissions

My prayer

Song by Julie Morsillo, 1983

May my life be a prayer
Journeying towards God
Wanting only to serve all
A discipline of love
A discipline of love

May my words be ever kind
Others to encourage
Careful not to criticise
But speak of good alone
Speak of good alone.

May my actions be always pure
Working for the common good
Striving for justice everywhere
Not hurting anyone
Not hurting anyone

May my heart be filled with love
Seeking purity of thought
Caring for all creation
With a spirit of joy
With a spirit of Joy
WITH A SPIRIT OF JOY.

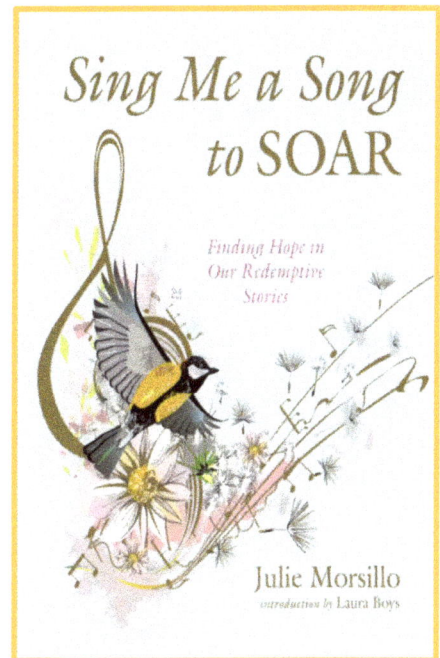

My prayer – previously published in author's first handbook in Dec 2024 – *Sing me a song to SOAR*

www.ingramcontent.com/pod-product-compliance
Lightning Source LLC
Chambersburg PA
CBHW061457270326
41931CB00021BA/3488